The FAT BURNER Diet

Patrick Holford & Bridget Woods

ION PRESS

First published in 1992
by ION Press, London.

Illustrations and cover: Christopher Quayle
Lay-out: Heather James

ISBN 1 870976 06 1

Printed and bound in Great Britain by
RAP Ltd, Rochdale
on recycled paper

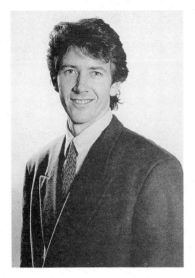

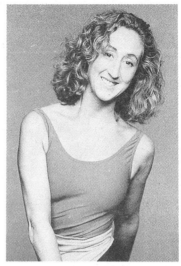

PATRICK HOLFORD started his career in the field of psychology. While studying at the University of York he researched the role of nutrition in mental health. His fascination with this subject led him to the US where he studied the work of leading figures in nutritional medicine. He has since researched into mental health, premenstrual syndrome, athletic performance and weight control. In 1984 he founded the Institute for Optimum Nutrition, an educational trust where he now teaches and practices.

He is Britain's leading nutritional author writing for a number of major national publications and frequently appearing on radio and television. His books include The Whole Health Manual, The Family Nutrition Workbook, Optimum Nutrition, and many others.

BRIDGET WOODS is one of Britain's pioneers in the field of fitness. In 1979 she brought aerobics to Britain, and, in 1981, held Britain's biggest aerobic work-out in Hyde Park. In 1983 she founded the Fitness Centre, London's largest and most progressive fitness club. Bridget spends her time between London and Los Angeles, helping her to introduce new ideas into her classes and private training sessions for the many celebrities with whom she works.

Now she has developed an innovative workout programme that will help you to burn fat, improve muscle tone and get you in shape - in fifteen minutes a day. Bridget's Fatburner exercises are also available on video.

She is fitness consultant to many national publications and frequently appears on television.

ACKNOWLEDGEMENTS

We would like to thank the many people who have helped create this book: Christopher Quayle, who designed the cover and took the photographs; Anne Pelter, for her help with the recipes; Kate Neil and Janet Anders for their technical support and proofing; and most of all, Heather James for her generous support, lay-out and design.

Guide to abbreviated measures

1 gram (g) = 1,000 milligrams (mg) = 1,000,000 micrograms (mcg)
Most vitamins are measured in milligrams or micrograms. Vitamins A, D and E are also measured in International Units (iu), a measurement designed to provide standardisation of the different forms of these vitamins that have different potencies.

1mcg of retinol or 2mcg of beta carotene = 3.3iu of vitamin A
1mcg of vitamin D = 40iu
1mg of vitamin E = approx. 1iu of d-alpha tocopherol
1 pound (lb) = 16 ounces (oz)   2.2lbs = 1 kilogram (kg)
In this book calories means kilocalories (kcals)

2 teaspoons (tsp) = 1 dessertspoon (dsp)
3 teaspoons (tsp) = 1 tablespoon (tbsp)
1.5 dessertspoons = 1 tablespoon (tbsp)
5 ml = 1 teaspoon
10 ml = 1 dessertspoon
15 ml = 1 tablespoon

References

Many references from respected scientific literature have been referred to in this book. A full list of these references, listed for each chapter, is available from the Institute for Optimum Nutrition, 5 Jerdan Place, London, SW6 1BE. Please send £2 and an SAE.

CONTENTS

INTRODUCTION

Most diets say what you eat, less what you 'burn off' through exercise, ends up as a wadge of fat around your middle. The only way to slim, they tell us, is to eat less or exercise more. But why can some people eat masses and never put on weight, while others have to almost starve to avoid the pounds creeping on? The difference is your metabolism, put simply, your ability to burn fat.

Consider this simple experiment, carried out by the Sunday Times magazine. They selected two willing slimmers. One was put on the Cambridge Diet, supplying 330 calories a day. One was put on the Fatburner Diet, supplying around 1,500 calories a day. Each lost 10lbs in the month. However, two weeks later the Cambridge dieter had regained 5lbs. About the diet, she said "The first three days were torturous but from then on it got worse. I was constantly exhausted and couldn't concentrate so that my work suffered badly. I blew up like a balloon when I resumed eating, and seemed to retain gallons of water. When I first stopped the diet, irresistible bingeing took over but after six weeks, with the exercise of limbs and discipline, I've managed to limit the damage to a gain of 5lbs." The Fatburner Diet volunteer regained 2lbs and had this to say "After the first few days I began to feel wonderful - alert and fit and thoroughly detoxified, with no more puffy eyes staring back from the bathroom mirror."

Conventional calorie theory cannot explain the difference in these results. How could a diet supplying three times the calories produce more weight loss with less suffering? After working with slimmers for over a decade I have become convinced that the secret to successful slimming lies not in calorie counting, but in improving the body's ability to burn fat. Hundreds of satisfied slimmers bear testimony to this.

For example, Rosemary weighed 10 stone and wanted to weigh 9 stone. Four months later she did. At her follow-up consultation she said "I've been on diets all my life. I found losing weight on this diet surprisingly easy. I thought Christmas would be difficult, but it wasn't. I don't want to eat as I did before." Hilary lost 2 stone and 8lbs over six months and with it she lost her low energy, her premenstrual problems, her frequent headaches and bad skin. "I have never felt hungry on this diet." she told me "I'll never go back to eating like I used to." Like the vast majority of my clients her loss of weight and well-being were still improving one year later.

In 1987 fatburning was put to the test when my book, The Metabolic Diet, was published. Three magazines selected volunteers to put this diet to the test. This is what they said:

"The diet proved such a success with readers that we decided to put three people on the diet for three months and watch what happened. Ian went from 15 stone 5lbs to 14 stone and felt so good he gave up smoking. Sabine wanted to lose at least 7lbs and lost 10lbs. Her only problem was coping with the extra energy. Gina lost 10lbs and continues to lose 1 to 2lbs a week. All felt positively healthy on the diet."

Woman's Realm magazine

"Increased alertness was a significant benefit. By the third day, everybody felt well - alert on rising, and three of us (including me) were bounding about full of the joys of spring. Two out of ten felt hungry, but the rest said that, as far as hunger was concerned, it was a comparatively easy diet to stick to. Mrs Kilby noted by day four that her concentration had improved, and this was backed up by other testers. Nobody had that weak and wobbly feeling associated with dieting. By the end of the week, everyone had stayed the course. Weight loss varied from 3lbs to 7lbs, 4 to 5lbs being the average."

She Magazine

"Weight loss: 4 to 7lbs in four weeks
Verdict: makes you look and feel good
Side effects: None"

Time Out

Meanwhile, in Northern Ireland, a trial was under way comparing the effects of the fatburning approach, with Unislim, a weight loss system involving a low calorie diet plus regular support meetings. After three months the fatburners had lost, on average, 13.7lbs, while the Unislim dieters had lost only 2lbs. Even more impressive was the steady weight loss of around a pound a week for the fatburners, compared to rapid weight loss in the first month, followed by increasing weight gain in subsequent months for the Unislim dieters.

The Fatburner Diet is the modern approach to successful slimming. It is low in calories, (around 1,500 a day) but no so low that you'll go hungry. It contains exercise, (about 15 minutes a day) but not so much that you'll have difficulty sticking to it. But, most of all, it is based on the principle of improving your ability to burn fat by making the body more efficient. By eating the right quality of food as well as the right quantity, and by taking the right quality of exercise, as well as the right quantity slimming becomes so much easier.

A Diet For Life with Permanent Results

The Fatburner diet isn't just a diet to follow to lose weight. It's a way of life that will make you fit, healthy and lean. By the time you've reached your ideal weight you'll not only look good, you'll feel good too. Once you've felt the benefits you won't want to go back to your bad habits ever again. Unlike crash diets, as long as you stick to the basic principles, the pounds won't creep back on.

Part One of this book explains how fatburning works. **Part Two** shows you how to get fatburning now! **Part Three** teaches you the Fatburner exercise routine, with plenty of options depending on your lifestyle and temperament. **Part Four** shows you what to eat to burn fat, with many delicious recipes to tempt you.

PART ONE

How Fatburning Works

WHY DIETING DOESN'T WORK

C alorie counting diets say that what you eat, less what you 'burn off' through exercise, ends up as a wadge of fat around your middle. So if you want to lose weight what you have to do is eat less or exercise more. Simple, but is it right? In theory, but not in practice. Firstly, this approach does not embrace why we overeat (or under-exercise), and secondly it doesn't work. Consider this simple example. A banana is approximately 100 calories, so if you eat a banana less every day for a year you'd lose 36,500 calories. A pound of body fat is equivalent to around 4,000 calories. That means you'd lose 10 pounds in the first year, 3.5 stone by the fifth year, 7 stone after ten years and vanish completely after fifteen years! All by eating once less banana a day.

The calorie equation for exercise is equally ridiculous. Cycle vigourously for 15 minutes each day and you will lose 10lb in the first year. Quite Possibly. But 7 stone after ten years? No chance. However, according to calorie theory, a banana every day undoes all that hard work.

According to Dr.Michael Colgan, nutritionist to many Olympic athletes, some of his clients burn off over 7,000 calories a day, but eat only 3,500 calories. By calorie theory these athletes should have completely disappeared by now.

An investigation by Dr.Apfelbaum of people living in famine in the Warsaw ghetto during the second world war came up with the same contradiction. With an average calorie intake of 700 to 800 calories a day, and a requirement of around 2,500 calories, a deficiency of 1,241,000 calories would have built up over two years. The average body has 30 pounds of fat, representing 120,000 calories, to dispose of. Even if all the fat were lost, what happened to the remaining one million calories?

Metabolism is the Missing Link

The reason why calorie theory doesn't add up is the key to what's missing in most calorie controlled diets. The missing link is metabolism. Metabolism is the process of turning the fuel in food into energy that the body can use - and burning off unwanted fat. People vary considerably in their ability to turn food into energy and to burn fat. Those that don't do it well have a slow metabolism and consequently turn more food into fat. Most obese people have slower rates of metabolism than slim people. One of the big problems with crash diets below 1,000 calories is that the body sees this reduction in food as a threat and slows down the metabolic rate by as much as 45%. In the short term you can lose around 7lbs of body fluid and , if you're lucky, an absolute maximum of two pounds of body fat a week, which, together could account for as much as 10 pounds in two or three weeks. But the minute you go back to what you were eating before, the fluid returns, and so will the fat because your metabolic rate has slowed down, meaning that you now need less food to maintain a stable weight. Of course, this 'rebound effect' is good business for food replacement programmes, whose customers try crash dieting on average three times a year.

Consider the story of Michelle and Caroline, two volunteers for The Sunday Times Tried & Tested diet feature. Michelle was put on the Cambridge Diet, a 330 calories a day food replacement diet. Caroline was put on The Metabolic Diet, a 1,500 calorie diet used by the Institute for Optimum Nutrition that is based on influencing your metabolism rather than just reducing calories. According to Michelle "The first three days were torturous but from then on it got worse. Walking down the road required serious will: I was constantly exhausted and couldn't concentrate so that my work suffered badly. Weight loss came slowly - I'd expected miracles after reading the publicity boasts - but in the final week it finally plummeted. My face acquired the desired gaunt look... but unfortunately my bust rapidly followed suit. I blew up like a balloon when I resumed eating, and seemed to retain gallons of water; conversely, 'loose' skin has appeared, creating an under-arm bat-wing effect. When I first stopped the diet, irresistible bingeing took over but after six weeks, with the exercise of limbs

11

and discipline, I've managed to limit the damage to a gain of five pounds. " Michelle lost 10 lbs and gained 5. Caroline also lost ten lbs in a month and had put on 2 lbs on holiday after the diet. When asked about her diet she commented " One of the hardest, but best things about it was the insistence on giving up coffee and stimulants. I had caffeine withdrawal headaches for the first few days, but began to feel wonderful after that - alert and fit and thoroughly detoxified, with no more puffy eyes staring back from the bathroom mirror. I regained 2 lbs while on holiday but will whittle it off by eating sensibly. "

Very Low Calorie Diets Are Not The Answer

Food replacement programmes involving very low calorie diets rarely produce long-term weight loss any more effectively than the fatburner approach. Due to public concern about the safety of such diets very low calorie diets must now provide at least 400 calories per day for women and 500 calories per day for men, and at least 40 grams of protein for women and 50 grams of protein for men. The reason for this is that if you greatly limit your calorie intake the body must break down body fat or protein in order to make energy. Of course, the objective is to break down fat, but how can you be sure the body is not breaking down muscle tissue or even vital organs? By providing a sufficient amount of dietary protein the loss of body protein is unlikely. However, these food replacement programmes fail on two other counts. Firstly, they do not encourage re-education of eating habits so when participants come off the diet they are more likely to go back to the kind of foods they were eating before. Secondly, the body sees a very low calorie diet as starvation and consequently lowers metabolic rate to conserve itself, which includes the fat. Returning to a previously balanced diet, but with a lower metabolic rate, means extra weight gain.

The Fibre Fad

The problems with calorie theory aren't just mathematical. The major problem with strictly calorie controlled diets is that you get hungry. So, how can you follow a low calorie diet without starving? The answer was fibre. Riding on the back of the fibre boom, wheat fibre, or bran, a by product of refining wheat flour, has been promoted to a princely food, but partly for the wrong reason. Studies using increased quantities of dietary wheat fibre or fibre capsules have not reported effects on weight loss.

To test these approaches we put ten people on a 1,000 calorie diet plus high fibre for a period of three months. Four lasted the course, with an average weight loss of 3.25lbs. The high drop-out rate is a reflection of how difficult it is to stick to a low calorie diet for a long period of time. In another study we put ten slimmers on high fibre tablets claimed to induce weight loss, for a period of three months. Five completed the three months with an average weight loss of 1.5lbs.

Now, although the fibre boom still continues, low calorie high fibre diets have not proved to be the answer as far as weight loss is concerned.

Eat Fat, Grow Slim?

Advocates of high-fat, low carbohydrate diets believe that if you don't eat carbohydrate you must burn fat instead. Fat is, after all, a good form of fuel, giving twice as much energy per gram. But burning fat is a bit like lighting a log with a match - it doesn't work. You need kindling to get a good 'fat' fire burning and carbohydrate is the kindling. So just like a fire that smokes because it burns inefficiently, a high fat diet gives off smoke in the form of 'ketones'. High-fat advocates claim that this inefficient metabolism means a loss of potential fat calories as ketones are excreted. But other scientists beg to differ. Research has clearly established that, at the most, 100 to 150 kcals are lost in ketone excretion, and what is more worrying, excessive ketone levels are extremely dangerous.

High Protein Diets

High protein, low carbohydrate diets are also to be avoided for health reasons. By restricting calorie intake, inefficient fat breakdown may occur, again causing an increase in ketones. Protein may also be used for fuel, and the advocates of this approach argue that protein is hard to convert and therefore less calories are consumed by the body at the end of the day. There may be an element of truth in this, but any diet which aims to imbalance metabolism is at best a short-term answer and at worst positively bad for your health. After all, 58 deaths have been associated with low calorie, high protein diets.

No Fat Diets

Since most dieters are fat phobic no-fat diets have proven popular. These diets rule out any sources of dietary fat as the primary means of cutting down on calories. To that end they are effective. However, the danger with these diets is that essential fats may also be excluded. Essential fats, called EFAs (Essential Fatty Acids) are needed by the body to control hormone levels, including the production of sex hormones, inflammation, the health of the heart and arteries and also the skin. EFA deficiency is quite common even among people who are not on a fat-free diet so the chances of a fat-free regime increasing the risk of deficiency are high. EFAs are predominantly found in nuts, seeds and cold-pressed seed oils such as sesame and sunflower. They are not found in olive oil or most margarines.

Fasting Diets

Modified fasts are the most severe approach to dieting. For those with life-threatening obesity they may be of value, but they are certainly not for the average person. One study followed 207 patients hospitalized for fasting, over a nine year period. While 79 reduced their weight to within 30 per cent of their ideal weight, 90 per cent were back to their original weight nine years later. Hardly a long-term solution.

So now you know what doesn't work... what's the secret of getting your metabolism working for you rather than against you? How do you get your body to turn food into energy, rather than fat, and to burn off those unwanted pounds?

FACTOR ONE

THE FATBURNER DIET

Have you ever stopped to think what you're made of? You are quite literally what you eat. The protein, fat and carbohydrate you eat, and the water you drink, turns into you. The average human body is 62% water, 17% protein, 6% minerals, 1% carbohydrate and between 10 and 20% fat. The reason why a very small proportion of us consists of carbohydrate is because this is our major source of fuel. The body can derive energy from complex carbohydrates such as wholegrains, beans, lentils and vegetables much more efficiently than any other foods. If we take in more than we need it gets put into storage as fat.

Protein, on the other hand, is the building material for new cells. We make an extraordinary number of new cells every minute. For instance, in four days the lining of your entire digestive tract is renewed. In twenty days you effectively have a new skin! All this energy making and cell building is controlled by vitamins, minerals and essential fatty acids, EFAs for short. These we require in very small amounts.

Dietary fat, with the exception of these EFAs, is completely unnecessary. It is bad fuel but can be burnt for energy if necessary. Conversely, if we eat too much of any kind of food the excess can be converted to body fat.

The Fatburner Diet is based on giving the body exactly what it needs, no more, no less, so that it can most efficiently burn off unwanted fat, and turn food into energy instead of flab. It is founded on four principles.

● Balancing Your Diet

It isn't just the quantity, but the quality of what you eat that makes a difference to your weight. The first principle of the Fatburner Diet is to give your body the right balance of fat, protein and carbohydrate.

● Vitamin Vitality

The second principle is to ensure that you have an optimal intake of the catalysts: vitamins, minerals and EFAs, that allow the body's metabolism to work at its best. This is explained more fully in the next chapter. The foods we recommend in the Fatburner Diet are all rich in vitamin vitality.

● Balancing Your Blood Sugar

The complex carbohydrate you eat turns into glucose, a simple sugar, in the blood. Glucose is the form of fuel cells can burn. Keeping an even blood sugar level is critical to your appetite, energy and weight. Too much glucose in the blood and the excess turns to fat. Too little and you will feel tired and hungry. Simple, refined carbohydrates, which includes sugar, alcohol and refined foods, are not good because they short-cut the body's normal digestion processes and rush straight into the blood stream, sometimes causing a short-term boost to energy levels, but in the long-term contribute to weight gain. Stimulants, which include tea, coffee, chocolate and cigarettes, do the same thing and are best avoided or considerably reduced if you want to maintain an even weight.

● The Fibre Factor

Fibre helps to reduce appetite as well as having other health benefits. Most people think of bran when they think of fibre, but wheat bran is one of the least effective fibres. The fibres in vegetables, oats, lentils and beans are much more effective. As well as making food more bulky and therefore making you feel full, they also help to control blood sugar levels. Some types of vegetable fibre are so effective in controlling blood sugar levels that they are used in the treatment of diabetes.

● BALANCING YOUR DIET

The average diet derives 42% of calories from fat, 15% from protein and the remaining 43% from mainly refined carbohydrates and sugar. The ideal diet should derive no more than 30% of calories from fat, 15% from protein and the remaining 55% from mainly complex carbohydrates.

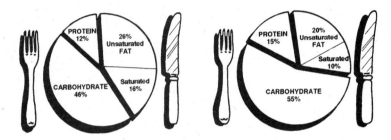

Figure 1   *The Average Diet vs The Optimum Diet*

So most of us need to cut down on our fat consumption (meat, dairy produce, fried foods and high fat spreads), our simple sugar consumption (from sweet snacks, drinks, added sugar and foods containing sugar) and increase complex carbohydrates. Simply doing this will cut down your calorie intake because complex carbohydrates are more filling and keep you satisfied for longer.

Protein Myths

Many people eat more protein than they need. If your body is working efficiently, which means having the right supply of vitamins and minerals which turn food protein into body protein, you need to eat less protein. If the kind of protein you eat is high quality, again you need less. The protein in eggs, dairy produce, fish, meat, rice, oats, seeds, and soya beans are all high quality. But how much of these foods are protein? Eggs, milk, rice and oats are less than 10% protein. This means that, even though the quality of protein is good, you'd still need to eat a lot to get enough protein. In the case of oats and rice the excess is mainly complex carbohydrate, so that would be fine. But milk and eggs are high in fat, so that would not be so good. Even lean meat is high in fat. A steak, for example, can derive as much as 70% of its calories from fat.

So, once again, it is both the quantity and quality that counts. The quality of protein in foods of vegetable origin can be increased by eating them in certain combinations. This is because the quality of protein depends on the balance of amino acids in the protein. In the same way that words are made out of letters, protein is made out of amino acids. The amino acids lacking in beans are plentiful in rice. The combination of the two produces a protein quality equivalent to eggs. Any of the combinations below increase the quality of protein. These don't have to be combined in the same meal, but should be eaten in the same day.

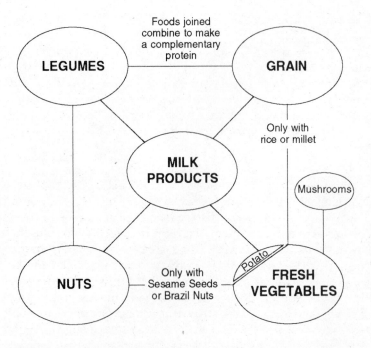

Figure 2 *Combining Foods for Higher Quality protein*

When the protein you eat is good quality, and your body is working well, the amount you need is less. Any two of the following would more than amply provide the average daily protein requirement, while being low in saturated fat. If food groups are combined smaller servings are required:

Lentils (uncooked) 1/3 cup (92g)
Tuna, canned 1 small tin (84g)
1 baked sardine
1 cup sunflower seeds (188g)
1 cup almonds (110g)
2 medium eggs (169g)
1 small pot cottage cheese (129g)
1 small lamb chop (110g)
1 small breast roast chicken (71g)
2.5 cups of rice (338g)
1 large tin of baked beans (430g)
0.5 cup of peanuts (90g)
1 cup of frozen peas (259g)
0.66 cup red kidney beans (99g)
0.66 cup chick peas (109g)
0.33 cups soya beans (200g)
3.5 oz cheddar cheese (84g)
2 cups of other beans (275g)
3 small pots natural yoghurt (440g)
1 packet of tofu (soya bean curd) (275g)
2 cups wheatgerm (132g)

Fat Facts

Not all fat is the same. Saturated fat is not essential for life, and eating too much is associated with a greater risk for heart disease and cancer as well as obesity. Saturated fats are solid at room temperature and include most of the fat found in butter, cream, cheese, margarine and meat. Unsaturated fats, or rather oils, since they are liquid at room temperature, are found mainly in nuts, seeds and fish. Certain kinds of unsaturated fats are now known to be essential for health, keeping hormones in balance, arteries healthy and helping to control inflammation hence alleviating conditions such as arthritis, asthma and eczema. These kinds of fats are called EFAs (essentail fatty acids). If your diet is low in fat overall and a high proportion of the fat you eat is EFAs this actually helps you to burn fat!

The Seeds of Life

EFAs are found in fish, nuts and seeds. They are converted in the body into complex substances that control many body functions. This conversion depends upon the presence of vitamin B6, magnesium and zinc. Conversely, too much alcohol, saturated fat, stress and smoking block this conversion.

The best sources of EFAs are fatty fish, sesame and sunflower seeds, or their oils. Olive oil does not contain EFAs. EFAs are easily destroyed by heat so its best to buy cold-pressed oil and use it in small amounts only for salad dressings, not for cooking. Spreads such as 'tahini', made from sesame seeds are also good sources. Sesame seeds themselves can be ground and sprinkled onto cereal, soups and other dishes. They are packed full of minerals and vitamin E as well.

Butter or Margarine?

Butter contains saturated fat. Margarine contains 'hydrogenated' polyunsaturated fat, which makes the fat solid, in other words saturated. This processed unsaturated fat is no better for you than butter and does not have the beneficial effects of EFAs. Some margarines add back a small amount of unprocessed nut or seed oil. This is why some margarines melt more easily than butter.

Low Fat not No Fat

We recommend you to avoid all concentrated sources of saturated fat, such as meat, high fat dairy produce and spreads. Grill or bake food instead or frying. On occasion foods can be sauteed, using a tiny amount of butter or olive oil, just to grease the pan. Once the ingredients are sizzling add in two tablespoons of water, vegetable stock, lemon juice or diluted soya sauce (depending on the recipe) to 'steam-fry' food. Do not, however, avoid nuts and seeds completely. Some of our recipes include sesame seeds, almonds and chestnuts, which are less fatty than sunflower seeds, brazils, walnuts and pecans.

Carbohydrates - How Complex Are They?

The human body is designed to run on complex carbohydrates which means wholegrains, beans, lentils and vegetables. The body can derive energy from these much more efficiently than any other foods. Fruit is an exception. Although classified as a simple carbohydrate it is not 'fast releasing' like sugar, because the fructose in fruit has to be converted in the liver into glucose before the body can use it. This slows down its release into the blood stream and also makes it a desirable fuel.

Mankind has, however, learnt how to cheat nature by isolating the sweetness in food and discarding the rest. All forms of concentrated sugar, white sugar, brown sugar, malt, glucose, honey and syrup are 'fast releasing' sugars, causing a rapid increase in blood sugar levels. The way the body responds to a rapid increase in blood sugar levels is to take the sugar into the cells. If they don't need it the sugar is turned into fat. Most concentrated forms of sugar are also devoid of vitamins and minerals, unlike their natural sources, such as fruit. Without vitamins and minerals metabolism becomes inefficient, again contributing to poor weight control.

However, it is not only concentrated forms of sugar that cause this problem. All over-cooked or over-processed carbohydrates become simple sugar. White and brown bread, white rice, cornflakes and instant mashed potato have as strong an effect on blood sugar as a Mars Bar.

● BALANCING YOUR BLOOD SUGAR

Keeping your blood sugar balanced is probably the most important factor in weight control. The level of glucose in your blood largely determines your appetite. When the level drops you feel hungry. The glucose in your bloodstream is available to body cells to make energy. When the levels are too high the body converts the excess to glycogen (a short term fuel store mainly in the liver and muscle cells) or fat, our long-term energy reserve. When the levels are too low we experience a whole host of symptoms including fatigue, poor concentration, irritability, nervousness, depression, excessive thirst, sweating, headaches and digestive problems. An estimated three in every ten people have glucose intolerance, an inability to keep an even blood sugar level. Their blood sugar level may go too high and then drop too low. The result, over the years, is that they become increasingly fat and lethargic. On the other hand, if you can control your blood sugar levels the result is even weight and constant energy.

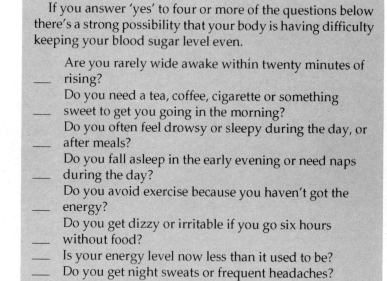

If you answer 'yes' to four or more of the questions below there's a strong possibility that your body is having difficulty keeping your blood sugar level even.

___ Are you rarely wide awake within twenty minutes of rising?

___ Do you need a tea, coffee, cigarette or something sweet to get you going in the morning?

___ Do you often feel drowsy or sleepy during the day, or after meals?

___ Do you fall asleep in the early evening or need naps during the day?

___ Do you avoid exercise because you haven't got the energy?

___ Do you get dizzy or irritable if you go six hours without food?

___ Is your energy level now less than it used to be?

___ Do you get night sweats or frequent headaches?

Figure 3 Glucose Tolerance Check

So what makes your blood sugar level unbalanced? Obviously eating too much sugar and sweet foods. However, the kind of foods that have the greatest effect are not always what you might expect. The chart overleaf shows which foods have the most profound effect on blood sugar levels. The worst is glucose which is the simplest form of sugar. Malt, sugar, Lucozade and Mars Bars all contain glucose, as does most honey. Fructose, the sugar in fruit, has little effect.

Of the fruits, bananas and dried fruit have the greatest effect on blood sugar, and apples have the least. Whole grains have a small effect on blood sugar, unless they are refined. Commercial bread, brown or white, white rice and white pasta all have increased effects compared to their whole counterparts. The best bread is Scandinavian whole rye grain bread, such as Pumpernickel bread. Oatcakes also have a small effect on blood sugar. Cornflakes came out badly for breakfast cereals, with porridge oats being the best.

The best foods of all are pulses - peas, beans and lentils. None of these have substantial effects on blood sugar. Milk products, which contain the sugar lactose, are also good. Surprisingly, even ice-cream comes out well. But don't kid yourself - it's still high in fat, even if it doesn't alter blood sugar levels much.

Vegetables, when cooked or highly processed, can have a considerable effect on blood sugar. Carrots and parsnips are the sweetest vegetables, however, if eaten raw or lightly cooked, have a much less dramatic effect.

Which Foods Raise Blood Sugar Levels?

The foods with the greatest effect on blood sugar have the highest score.

Sugars

Glucose	100
Maltose	100
Lucozade	95
Honey	87
Mars Bar	68
Sucrose (sugar)	59
Fructose	20

Fruit

Raisins	64
Bananas	62
Orange juice	46
Oranges	40
Apples	39

Grain Products

Brown bread	72
White rice	72
White bread	69
Ryvita	69
Brown rice	66
Pastry	59
Digestive biscuits	59
Sweetcorn	59
Rich tea biscuits	55
Oatmeal biscuits	54
White spaghetti	50
Wholemeal spaghetti	42

Cereals

Cornflakes	80
Weetabix	75
Shredded wheat	67
Muesli	66
All-Bran	52
Poridge oats	49

Pulses

Baked beans (no sugar)	40
Butter beans	36
Chick peas	36
Blackeye beans	33
Haricot beans	31
Kidney beans	29
Lentils	29
Soya beans	15

Dairy Products

Ice cream	36
Yoghurt	36
Whole milk	34
Skimmed milk	32

Vegetables

Cooked parsnips	97
Cooked carrots	92
Instant potato	80
New potato	70
Cooked beetroot	64
Peas	51

Figure 4 *Glyceamic Index of Foods*

Alcohol, which is a chemical cousin of sugar, also upsets blood sugar levels. So do stimulants, like tea, coffee, cola drinks, and cigarettes. These substances, like stress itself, stimulate the release of adrenalin and other hormones that initiate the "fight or flight" response. This prepares the body for action, by releasing sugar stores and raising blood sugar levels, to give our muscles and brain a boost of energy. Unlike our ancestors whose main stresses (like running up a tree to avoid being eaten for dinner) required a physical response, twentieth century stress is mainly mental or emotional. The body has to cope with the excess of blood sugar by releasing yet more hormones to take the glucose out of circulation. The combination of too much sugar, stimulants and prolonged stress taxes the body and results in an inability to control blood sugar levels, which, if severe enough, can develop into diabetes.

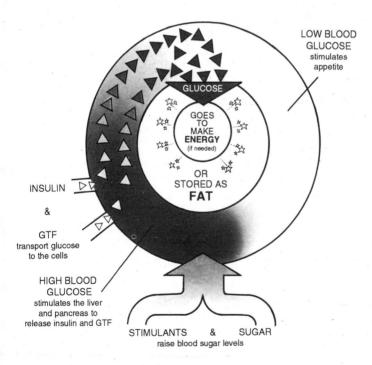

Figure 5 *The Sugar Cycle*

The only way out of this vicious cycle is to reduce or avoid all forms of concentrated sweetness, tea, coffee, alcohol and cigarettes, and start eating foods that help to keep your blood sugar level even. The best foods are all kinds of beans, peas and lentils, oats and wholegrains. These foods are high in complex carbohydrates and contain special factors that help release their sugar content gradually. They are also high in fibre which helps normalise blood sugar levels.

●THE FIBRE FACTOR

High fibre diets are definitely recommended for general health reasons. Those on high fibre diets have less risk of bowel cancer, diabetes or diverticular disease, and are unlikely to suffer from constipation.

Fibre is a natural constituent of a healthy diet high in fruits, vegetables, lentils, beans and wholegrains. There should be no need to add extra fibre if these foods are eaten. Professor Dickerson, formerly Head of Nutrition at the University of Surrey has stressed the danger of adding wheat bran to a nutrient-poor diet. The reason for this is that wheat bran contains high levels of phytates, which reduce the absorption of essential minerals, including zinc.

Fibre is calorie free and there is little doubt that a diet high in naturally occurring fibre is more satisfying. After all, which would you find easier to eat: two sweet biscuits, or a pound of carrots? Each have the same calories.

One of the main reasons why high fibre foods are more satisfying is that fibre absorbs water and therefore foods containing fibre become bulkier in the digestive tract. About 10 litres of digestive juices are released every day into the digestive tract, so the ability of the food you eat to absorb this water would make a big difference to the bulk of material being digested. Wheat fibre, as in bran, is not very absorbent compared to some vegetable fibres. While wheat fibre placed in water will swell to ten times its original volume, the fibre from the Japanese konjac plant, for example, swells to 100 times its volume. Of the grain fibres, the fibre in oats is the best in this respect and is therefore included in the Fatburner Diet.

Glucomannan Fibre

Konjac fibre, known as glucomannan, is one of many fibres that also help to control blood sugar balance. These fibres help to slow down the release of sugars within food into the blood stream. Overall, glucomannan fibre is undoubtedly the best fibre and has been used in the treatment of weight loss, constipation and diabetes. We tested the effects of a daily intake of 3 grams of glucomannan on ten overweight people over a three month period. Nine completed the trial, with an average weight loss of 6.6lbs each, with no apparent change to diet or exercise. Our results confirmed those of other researchers.

Thanks to a quirk in a new food law glucomannan extracted from konjac fibre is no longer permitted for sale in the UK, however konjac fibre is. Konjac fibre contains about 60 per cent glucomannan so a daily intake of 5 grams would be equivalent to 3 grams of glucomannan. We recommend the inclusion of konjac fibre for those wanting maximum weight loss.

FACTOR TWO

FATBURNING VITAMINS

Your ability to control your weight doesn't only depend on the kind of food, and the quantity you eat. It also depends on the vitamins and minerals in your diet, because these help every single cell in your body to turn food into energy, and to burn off unwanted fat. Any lack of these vital nutrients will result in less energy and consequently a greater predisposition to lay down fat.

How To Make Energy

The human body is made out of cells. The brain, muscles, liver, skin, immune system, heart and arteries are all simply a collection of cells. These cells do work for the body, whether it's digesting, thinking, or moving. The fuel for all cells is glucose derived from carbohydrate foods. So keeping an even blood sugar level, which is the fuel reserve for cells, is the first step in making energy.

Turning Glucose into Energy, instead of Fat

Within each of our thirty trillion or so cells exist tiny energy factories called mitochondria. The mitochondria turn glucose into another chemical, pyruvic acid , in the process of which a small amount of energy is released, which can be used by the cell to carry out its work. If this step occurs without sufficient oxygen present, a by-product builds up called lactic acid. That's why the first time you do strenuous exercise using muscles you didn't even know you had, the next day your muscles ache. This is, in part, because you've made them work too hard without supplying enough oxygen, causing a build up of lactic acid. The more you exercise, developing larger muscles, the less strain you put on the muscles and the more oxygen they can use. This is what aerobic exercise is all about - providing muscles cells with enough oxygen so they can work properly.

Pyruvic acid then gets turned into acetyl-coenzyme A, or A-coA for short. This substance is perhaps the most vital because if you're starved of glucose, for example when a marathon runner "hits the wall", you can break down fat or protein to AcoA, and use this for energy. However it's rather inefficient so the body prefers to use carbohydrate for fuel.

From this point on, oxygen is needed every step of the way. AcoA enters a series of chemical reactions known as the Krebs cycle, after its discover Ernst Krebs, which separates off hydrogen molecules, which then meet oxygen and, step by step, energy is released. In fact over 90 per cent of all our energy is derived in this final stage. The waste products are carbon dioxide, which we exhale, water, which goes to form urine, and heat. That's why you get hot when exercising, because muscle cells make lots of energy, so heat is created.

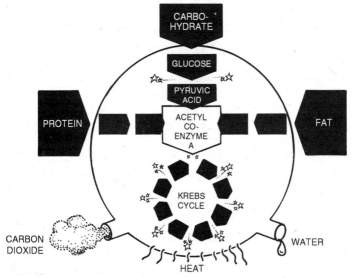

Figure 6 How Food Turns Into Energy

Fatburning Nutrients

If you're thinking all you need to do is eat complex carbohydrates and keep breathing that's only half the story. All these chemical reactions are carefully controlled by enzymes, themselves dependent on no less than eight vitamins and five minerals. Any shortage of these critical catalysts and your energy factories, the mitochondria, go out of tune. The result is inefficient energy production, a loss of stamina, highs and lows - or just lows.

The important vitamins are the B complex vitamins, a family of eight different substances, every one essential for making energy. Glucose can't be turned into pyruvic acid without B1 and B3 (niacin). AcoA can't be formed without B1, B2, B3, and most important of all, B5 (pantothenic acid). The Krebs cycle needs B1, B2 and B3 to do its job properly. Proteins and fats can't be used to make energy without B6, B12, folic acid and biotin.

Vitamins for Vitality

It used to be thought that as long as you ate a reasonable diet you'd get enough B vitamins. But studies have shown that long-term slight deficiencies gradually result in a depletion of these vitamins in cells, causing early warning signs of deficiency such as poor skin condition, anxiety, depression, mental confusion, irritability, but most of all, fatigue. Many people's diets fall short on these vital vitamins. The Booker Survey in 1985 showed that only one in ten people ate a diet that provided the Recommended Daily Allowance for B6 or folic acid. In one study at the Institute for Optimum Nutrition a group of 82 volunteers, many of whom already had a "well balanced diet" were assessed to calculate their optimal nutritional needs. All 82 were given extra B vitamins in supplement form, often in doses twenty times that of the RDAs. After six months 79 per cent of participants reported a definite improvement in energy, 61 per cent felt physically fitter, and 60 per cent had noticed an improvement in their mental alertness and memory.

Being water soluble, B vitamins are easily lost when foods are boiled in water, as well as being extremely sensitive to heat. The best natural sources are therefore fresh fruit, raw vegetables, and wheatgerm. Seeds, nuts and wholegrains contain reasonable amounts, as do meat, fish, eggs and dairy produce. But these levels are reduced when the food is cooked or stored for a long time.

The minerals iron, calcium, magnesium, chromium and zinc are also vital for making energy. Calcium and magnesium are perhaps the most important because all muscle cells need an adequate supply of these to be able to contract and relax. A shortage of magnesium, so common in those who don't eat much fruit or vegetables, often results in muscle cramps, as the muscle is unable to relax.

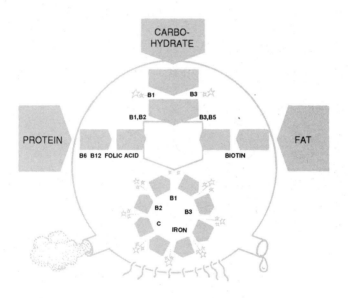

Figure 7 *Vitamins and Minerals Needed to Turn Food Into Energy*

Vitamin B3 and B6, and the minerals zinc and chromium are especially important because they help to supply fuel to cells, ready for burning. B6 and zinc are needed to make the enzymes that digest food. They are also essential in the production of the hormone insulin, which helps to control blood sugar levels. A lack of zinc also disturbs appetite control and causes a loss of sense of taste or smell, often leading to over-consumption of meat and cheese and other strong tasting foods.

Vitamin B3 and chromium are part of a vital substance produced in the liver, called 'glucose tolerance factor'. This, like insulin, helps to take glucose from the blood into cells, and helps keep an even blood sugar level.

The Myth of the Well Balanced Diet

Even if you eat the kind of foods we recommend you are unlikely to take in the amounts of vitamins and minerals needed to guarantee your metabolism is as efficient as possible. This may come as a surprise since we have been led to believe that "as long as you eat a well-balanced diet you get all the vitamins and minerals you need". However, the sad truth is that this is a lie. Every single survey in the past decade has shown that people who think they eat a well balanced diet are unlikely to meet all recommended daily intakes of vitamins and minerals.

These recommended intakes, called RDAs or RDIs, are themselves only designed to prevent certain deficiency diseases. They are certainly not optimal levels which are often many times higher and depend upon an individual's lifestyle, diet, health history and a host of other factors.

Deficiency is Widespread

Why are we so deficient? First of all, we choose the wrong foods. Two thirds of the average diet comes from refined flour, sugar and fat, all devoid of vitamins and minerals. The refining and processing of food often removes as much as 80 per cent of the nutrients present. For example, refining flour causes 98 per cent of chromium and 78 per cent of zinc to be lost. However, even wholesome food is not as 'whole' as it used to be. Some oranges contain no vitamin C! A 100g serving of wholewheat flour can provide as little as 0.3mg of vitamin B5, a fraction of the optimal intake of 50 to 100mg. Sometimes, these low levels result from losses due to storage. Food we eat today is obviously not as fresh as that of our jungle dwelling ancestors. Modern farming practices also have a lot to answer for.

We get our nutrients from plants, or from animals that have eaten plants. Plants make vitamins, provided they get the right elements, including minerals, from the soil. The minerals in the soil come from rocks being crushed during ice ages, volcanoes or other geological events. So there is a limited supply of minerals in the soil.

Modern farming methods have allowed us to over-farm the earth, to maximise food production and profit, without putting anything back. To make matters worse chemical fertiliser contains chemicals which bind up minerals like zinc and stop them being taken up by plants. Pollution, such as acid rain, has the same effect. Since many of these depleted minerals don't effect the growth of plants, only its nutritional value, farmers have no reason to remineralise the soil. For these reasons a carrot today is nothing like a carrot eaten by your ancestors, even though it may be the same colour and shape. Food grown by organic methods, which avoids the use of chemical fertilizers and adds minerals back into the soil, consequently have a higher nutrient content.

Calcium	60.0%
Phosphorous	70.9%
Magnesium	84.7%
Potassium	77.0%
Chromium	98.0%
Manganese	85.8%
Iron	75.6%
Zinc	77.7%
Selenium	15.9%
Molybdenum	48.0%

Figure 8 Minerals lost in refining flour

Fatburning Supplements

We recommend you to supplement your well-balanced diet with fatburning vitamins and minerals to ensure your metabolism is working at peak efficiency. The ideal intake is different for every individual and can be worked out individually for you by a nutrition consultant (see page 155). However, the chart below gives a good approximation of the optimal levels for an average person to supplement on top of a well balanced diet.

Vitamin		Optimum Daily Intake
Vitamin A	(retinol)	7,500iu
Vitamin B1	(thiamine)	75mg
Vitamin B2	(riboflavin)	75mg
*Vitamin B3	(niacin)	100mg
Vitamin B5	(pantothenate)	75mg
Vitamin B6	(pyridoxine)	100mg
Vitamin B12	(cobalamine)	10mcg
Folic Acid		100mcg
Biotin		50mcg
Vitamin C	(ascorbic acid)	1,000mg
Vitamin D	(califerol)	400iu
Vitamin E	(d-alpha tocopherol)	100iu

Mineral	Optimum Daily Intake
Calcium	200mg
Magnesium	100mg
Iron	10mg
Zinc	15mg
Manganese	5mg
Chromium	120mcg

*Niacin can cause a blushing sensation, especially if taken without food. This effect decreases with use and is not harmful. It is, in fact, beneficial and helps to remove cholesterol.

These levels are easily supplied by taking one or two supplement formulas. Most health food shops can help you to meet these levels in the simplest and least expensive way, choosing from a variety of good brands. One product which meet these levels particularly well is Health+Plus' *Metabolic Pack*.

The Health+Plus *Metabolic Pack* was formulated on the basis of our research and meets all these levels. The *Metabolic Pack* consists of a daily sachet of five supplements. (See page 155 for supply details.) These supplements cost as little as 35p a day, which is equivalent to three cigarettes, a bar of chocolate, a packet of crisps, or a cup of coffee.

Supplements should be taken with food, preferably with breakfast, or spread out throughout the day, since it is during the day that we make most energy and hence need a good supply of these nutrients. We recommend you to take them regularly, every day for at least three months.

FACTOR THREE

FATBURNING EXERCISES

The good news about exercise is that you really don't have to be fanatically fit to lose weight. And the reason why is not calories, it's metabolism.

According to calorie theory, exercise doesn't do much to promote weight loss. After all, running a mile only burns up 300 calories. That's equivalent to two slices of toast or a piece of apple pie. But this argument misses three key points.

1   **The effects of exercise are accumulative.** OK, so running a mile a day only burns up 300 calories, but if you do that three days a week for a year, that's 22,000 calories, equivalent to a weight loss of 11 pounds! Also, the amount of calories you burn up depends on how fat and fit you are to start with. The fatter and less fit you are the more benefit you'll derive from small amounts of exercise.

2   **Moderate exercise decreases your appetite.** A degree of physical activity is necessary for appetite mechanisms to work properly. Those who do not exercise have exaggerated appetites and hence the pounds gradually creep on.

3   **Exercise boosts your metabolic rate.** The most important reason why exercise is a key to weight loss is its effect on your metabolic rate. According to Professor McArdle, exercise physiologist at City University, New York, "Most people can generate metabolic rates that are eight to ten times above their resting value during

sustained cycling, running or swimming. Complementing this increased metabolic rate is the observation that vigourous exercise will raise metabolic rate for up to 15 hours after exercise."

Fatburner Exercises Boost Metabolism

Combining diet and exercise is the best way to lose weight. Weight lost through restrictive dieting is often half fat, half lean tissue, such as muscle. Since muscle burns up more energy (calories) than fat, the less muscle you have the slower is your metabolism. Combining the Fatburner Diet and the Fatburner exercise programme makes sure you lose fat, not lean muscle.

The Fatburner exercises improve metabolism. Brisk walking, jogging, cycling, swimming, aerobic dance, stepping, cross-country skiing, the Fatburner Air-obic circuit or any aerobic exercise that is steady and continuous and of a certain intensity will help to burn fat efficiently.

The Fatburner exercises also tone the body, reduce the risk of osteoporosis, increase muscle tissue, and reduce one's body fat percentage (high ratios of body fat to lean tissue have been linked to heart disease, diabetes and some cancers). These exercises will strengthen your heart and lungs, reduce your risk of heart disease, help control stress, and improve circulation. There are so many benefits of exercise, you may wonder why you haven't started sooner.

Fatburner Exercises Prevent Osteoporosis

Women, as they get older, are at a greater risk of developing osteoporosis, which can be a very painful, debilitating and sometimes underestimated disease. Osteoporosis causes gradual bone loss and brittleness. The best prevention is to develop the highest possible bone mass and maintain it. Proper nutrition, including enough calcium, and resistance training is the best way to do this. Bones need regular resistance in order to stay strong. Weightlessness studies at NASA have found that in the absence of gravity, bones begin to deteriorate. Just walking around stresses muscles and strengthens bones to some degree. So do everyday physical activities like carrying groceries.

You Don't Have To be Fanatically Fit

You do not have to be fanatically fit to embark on this programme. The important thing to remember is to stay within your training zone for your age (Part Three explains how to work out your training zone). An overweight, out of condition person may reach his or her training heart rate zone by walking just a few hundred yards, whereas a fitter, leaner person may have to walk briskly for at least five minutes to push their pulse up to their training zone. This is why we recommend you monitor your pulse while exercising to make sure you do not over push your body but push hard enough to get the fatburning benefits. As you get fitter and leaner you will find you will have to push harder, i.e., walk faster or add more hill walking to your programme.

Unfanatical Fitness Decreases Your Appetite

Contrary to popular belief, moderate exercise actually decreases your appetite. According to new evidence on appetite research, both animals and man consistently show decreased appetite with small increases in physical activity. One study looked at an industrial population in West Bengal, India. Those doing sedentary work ate more and consequently weighed more than those doing light work. As the level of work increased from light to heavy, workers ate more, but not relative to their energy output. The result was that the heavier the work, the lighter the worker.

About the Fatburner Exercises

There are two main elements to the Fatburner exercise programme.

The first element is **aerobic exercise** that will increase your metabolism and burn calories while you are exercising; the second element, **toning exercises** that will increase your percentage of lean muscle tissue. Lean muscle tissue is more metabolically active than fat. Therefore the higher muscle to fat ratio you have in your body, the higher your metabolic rate will be.

That is why two people of the same weight do not always burn up the same amount of calories, i.e., a 9-stone woman with a low body fat percentage may eat like a horse and not put on any weight, while her friend, another 9-stone woman, may just look at food and she will put on weight. Because she has a high body fat percentage, her ability to burn up calories is far lower than her friend with the low body fat percentage.

Lean tissue is more metabolically active than fat. Simply put, eight pounds of muscle burns more calories than eight pounds of fat. So it makes sense to perform exercises that will tone your muscles and improve your metabolic rate. The Fatburner Air-obic circuit does just that. It helps you to burn calories while you are exercising and will improve your muscle tone so that you will be able to burn calories even at rest.

By the time most people reach their 20's, their metabolic rate is already dropping. If you are inactive and do not continue strengthening the muscles in the body, you could lose an average of 1.5lbs of muscle each year after the age of 25. Muscles consume energy, thereby keeping your metabolic rate at a higher level so that your body stores fewer calories as fat. If your muscles are well conditioned and used frequently, they will burn calories around the clock, even while you are resting or sleeping.

Choosing Your Exercise

There are various forms of aerobic exercise available. The three we recommend are brisk walking, swimming and the Fatburner Air-obic Circuit. There are other alternatives, such as running, skipping, tennis, squash, football and basketball. The pros and cons of these exercises are discussed more fully in Part Three.

Increasing Your Activity Level

The good news is that you can double your energy output without doing any exercise as such. How? By increasing your baseline level of activity. Your baseline activity is the amount of energy you use up just going about your normal life. You can double this in a hundred different ways. For example, use the stairs instead of lifts. Walk the last mile to work. Even chopping vegetables rather than eating already prepared convenience food will give you more exercise! A study on six overweight men induced a 12.5lb weight loss in four months simply by walking 90 minutes a day, five days a week. This means that you could expect to lose 14lbs in a year just by walking the last 15 minutes to work and back. Every little bit counts.

How to Increase Your Baseline Activity

The Fat Way	The Fit Way
Take a lift	Use the stairs
Drive to work	Walk or cycle some of the way
Drive to the shops	Walk to the shops
Buy convenience foods	Cook fresh foods
Spend the night watching TV	Take up an active hobby
Get other people to bring you drinks	Get up and do it yourself (and get them one too!)
Use powered tools for gardening or DIY work	Use manual tools when it's just as quick
Go upstairs as little as possible at home	Run upstairs as often as possible
Use automatic car washes	Wash it yourself
Stick children in front of TV	Actively play with them
Have business meetings inside	Go for a walk where possible

How Hard Should I Exercise?

In order to achieve the fatburning benefits of exercise, you must raise your heart rate to a higher rate than normal. Your training heart rate zone is the level at which you should be working to efficiently burn fat as fuel. If you exercise at too high an intensity, you will start to work out anaerobically and your fuel source will change. You will also be increasing your risk of injury. If you exercise at too low an intensity, you will not be reaping the fat-burning benefits either. In Part Three you can find out what your Training Heart Rate Zone is, and how to measure it.

How Much Exercise Do I Need To Do?

If you follow the Fatburner exercise programme you need do as little as 15 minutes a day, in order to lose weight and gain shape. That's equivalent to 21 minutes of exercise, five days a week, giving yourself two days off. Alternatively, you may choose to 'double up' and exercise three times a week. It doesn't sound that difficult, does it? It isn't. Part Three tells you everything you need to know about fatburning exercise.

PART TWO

Get Fatburning Now!

GET FATBURNING NOW!

The Fatburner Diet is incredibly straightforward. In essence, all you have to do is:

- Eat any Fatburner recommended breakfast, lunch or dinner, plus two pieces of fresh fruit.
- Take the Fatburner recommended supplement programme every day.
- Do the Fatburner exercise routine.
- Stay off the AVOID foods and drinks and cut down the LIMIT food and drinks.

It's as simple as that!

Unlike other diets you may have been on you don't have to starve. According to Hilary Evans "I have never felt hungry on this diet" and she lost three stone. You don't have to suffer in order to slim. Quite the contrary. Most people feel more energised and alert within days of starting the Fatburner Diet.

Getting Started - The First Month

To make life even easier for you we've planned out an exact regime for you to follow for the first month. We recommend you **follow this regime strictly for the first month** for the following reasons: you'll get used to cooking and preparing the kinds of foods that are good for you; you'll get used to the kind of quantities you need; you'll break the habits that are stopping you losing weight; you'll get used to regular exercise and find a place for it in your daily schedule; as your energy increases and your weight and waist decrease nothing will stop you from going on.

Change is stressful. It's a natural reaction to resist change to your diet or your lifestyle, even when the change is for your own good. No doubt you'll have your resistances to the Fatburner Diet too. These are like old 'tapes' that run through your mind. "I bet this diet won't work", "I never stick to exercise regimes", "I don't have the will power", "I've got to have a bar of chocolate", "I'll never stick to this". Whatever your 'tapes' are, just recognise them as a string of words that run through your mind (repeatedly). You don't have to obey them. Whatever your resistance or your skepticism, **follow this regime strictly for the first month.** The results will speak for themselves.

Month Two and Three

After the first month, if its easier for you, you can just follow the "do's and don'ts", and adapt the recipes as you choose. Obviously, make sure the quantity you eat doesn't creep up, or the AVOID or LIMIT foods don't creep in. If you're the sort of person who would be likely to 'cheat' then follow the regime strictly, sticking to the recipes for the second and third month.

After Month Three

By the time you've been on the Fatburner Diet for three months you won't want to go back to eating like you used to. This regime will become a way of life, with all the long-term benefits of a good diet and regular exercise. When you reach your target weight it is still good to continue with this basic regime. You can, however, afford to be less strict with yourself. The Fatburner Diet is a diet for a long and healthy life, not just a diet to lose pounds and inches.

Here are the foods and drinks to increase, limit or avoid. If you're addicted to any 'avoid' foods or drinks or would find the limits unbelievably difficult, follow the tips on breaking your addiction. Use the first week of the diet to wean yourself off and find suitable alternatives.

INCREASE

These foods are generally low in fat and high in nutrients and can be eaten freely. They should form the major part of your diet.

All vegetables
All fresh fruits
All pulses which includes lentils, beans and peas
Low fat soya products such as tofu
Chestnuts
White fish
Wholegrain products
Oats, oat cakes, rice cakes
Skimmed milk
Diluted fruit juices
Herb teas, such as *Blackcurrant Bracer, Orange Dazzler, Apple Magic*
Coffee alternatives, such as *Caro* or *Caro Extra*
Water

LIMIT

These foods are best kept to a minimum. Some of these are included in the recipes in specific amounts because they contain important nutrients. However, some are also high in fat so do not have more than the recommended amounts.

Dried fruit
Nuts - except chestnuts
Coconut
Seeds
Salad dressings
Avocados
Vegetable oil and butter
Tahini and other spreads
Sugar-free jams
Bread, except wholegrain breads such as pumpernickel or 100% rye bread
Fatty fish such as herring, mackerel, tuna, kippers
Chicken, without skin
Game
Low fat cheese such as cottage cheese, Edam or Gouda
Whole milk and yoghurts
Eggs
Tea and coffee
Alcohol

AVOID

These foods are high in fat and are best strictly avoided during your weight loss programme. Once you have attained your target weight they may be eaten on occasion.

High fat meats including beef, pork, lamb, sausages and processed meats
Lard, dripping, suet and gravy
Deep fried food
Cream, ice cream and high fat cheeses
(Stilton, Cheddar, Cream Cheese)
High fat spreads and mayonnaises
Rich sauces made with cream or eggs
All sweets including chocolate
Sugar and foods with added sugar
Pastries, cakes and biscuits
Snack foods such as crisps

WEEK ONE - GETTING STARTED

There are quite a few changes you'll have to make to your diet and lifestyle to effectively lose weight, and change is never easy. We recommend you spend the first week getting yourself, and your kitchen, ready. Here's how.

Remove The Temptations

Start by using up or throwing away any AVOID foods in your fridge or larder. This is a great time to have people round for dinner! Restock your kitchen with the recommended foods and drinks. Do the same at work.

Vital Supplies

Some of the foods used in these recipes may be new to you. All of them are readily available in either your local health food shop, supermarket or the greengrocer's. Now that your fridge and larder are empty, fill them up with the recommended foods and drinks. Here's a list to help you get started.

WEEK One:

Rolled oats and oatflakes
Wheatgerm
Skimmed milk
Very low fat live yoghurt
Tofu
Honey
Raisins, dried apricots
Sunflower seeds
Mixed nuts, cashews, almonds, walnuts
Free range eggs
vanilla essence
Vegetable stock eg Vecon

Fruit: Apples, bananas, pears, oranges, raspberries, gooseberries, rhubarb, blackcurrants

Vegetables: Mushrooms, celery, spring onions, avocado, parsley, carrots, bean sprouts, potatoes, peppers, onions, garlic, cucumber, lettuce

Cheese: Cottage cheese, low fat quark or fromage frais, low fat cheddar cheese

Tuna fish in brine
Tamari
Brown rice
Tinned pineapple chunks
Rye or pumpernickel bread
Tahini
Cider vinegar
Olive oil, cold pressed
Very low fat mayonnaise
Chick peas, beans, lentils
White fish,
Tinned tomatoes or puree
Wholemeal flour
Wholemeal lasagne and wholemeal or buckwheat spaghetti
Bulgar (cracked wheat)

Drinks: Herb teas, such as Blackcurrant Bracer, Orange Dazzler, Apple Magic
Caro or Caro Extra
Get Up and Go
Aqua Libra

FOR OTHER WEEKS

Edam or Gouda
Fresh vegetables and fresh fruit
Millet
Oat cakes and rice cakes
Alfalfa seeds or sprouts
Couscous

Breaking Your Addictions

We recommend you greatly reduce your intake of stimulants such as tea, coffee, sugar, chocolate and alcohol. Here are some tips to help you break your addictions.

Coffee contains three stimulants - caffeine, theobromine and theophylline. Although caffeine is the strongest, theophylline is known to disturb normal sleep patterns and theobromine has a similar effect to caffeine, although it is present in much smaller amounts in coffee. So decaffeinated coffee isn't stimulant free.

A lot of coffee is definitely bad for you. High coffee consumers have a greater risk for cancer of the pancreas and a higher incidence of birth defects. Coffee also stops vital minerals being absorbed. The amount of iron absorbed is reduced to one third if coffee is drunk with a meal.

More controversial are the effects of small amounts of coffee. As a nutritionist I have seen many people cleared of minor health problems such as tiredness and headaches just from stopping drinking two or three coffees a day. The best way to find out what effect it has on you is to quit for a trial period of two weeks. You may get withdrawal symptoms for up to three days. These reflect how addicted you've become. After that, if you begin to feel perky and your health improves that is a good indication that you're better off without coffee. The most popular alternatives are Caro or Caro Extra, made with roasted barley, chicory and rye.

Tea is the great British addiction. A strong cup of tea contains as much caffeine as a weak cup of coffee and is certainly addictive. Tea also contains tannin which interferes with the absorption of vital minerals such as iron and zinc. Like coffee, drinking too much tea is also associated with a number of health problems including an increased risk of stomach ulcers. Particularly addictive is Earl Grey tea containing bergamot, itself a stimulant. If you're addicted to tea and can't get going without a cuppa it may be time to stop for two weeks and see how you feel. The best tasting alternatives are herb teas such as Blackcurrant Bracer, Orange Dazzler, Apple Magic or Raspberry Rendezvous. Drinking very weak tea irregularly is unlikely to be a problem.

Sugar is perhaps the most common addiction of all. The more sweet foods you have the greater your taste for sweetness. We all have a natural sweet tooth which is nature's way of attracting animals to eat fruits. In nature, sweet foods are usually safe to eat. But by refining sugar we've learnt how to cheat nature and eat the pure stuff. Nowadays concentrated sugar comes in many disguises - glucose, such as Lucozade, malt, honey or syrups. All these help to develop a sweet tooth, as do any food with concentrated sweetness, including grape juice or too much dried fruit such as raisins. However the sugar in most fruit, called fructose, does not have the same effect on the body as glucose, maltose or sucrose, which is normal sugar.

While too much sugar is associated with heart disease, diabetes, tooth decay and obesity, sugar is addictive because of its effect on energy and mood. Eating concentrated sources of sugar increases your blood sugar level giving more mental and physical energy, at least in the short term. This is one cause for hyperactivity, both in children and adults. If you're not aware of this effect it is most noticeable if you stay off sugar for two weeks then have a sugar binge.

Frequent over use of sugar can lead to glucose intolerance, which means an abnormal blood sugar balance. The symptoms may include irritability, aggressive outbursts, nervousness, depression, crying spells, dizziness, fears and anxiety, confusion, forgetfulness, inability to concentrate, fatigue, insomnia, headaches, palpitations, muscle cramps, excess sweating, digestive problems, allergies, blurred vision, excessive thirst and lack of sex drive. Does this sound like anyone you know? Probably three in every ten people have a mild form of glucose intolerance.

Kicking the sugar habit takes time and perseverance. It is best to wean yourself off slowly since your taste buds get used to less and less sweetness. Stop adding sugar to cereals, or eating cereals containing sugar, and add fruit instead. When you want something sweet have a piece of fresh fruit. Get used to diluting fruit juices with water. Gradually decrease your overall intake of sweet foods. Once you're basically sugar-free the odd sweet food is no big deal.

Chocolate is full of sugar. It also contains cocoa as its major active ingredient. Cocoa provides significant quantities of the stimulant theobromine, whose action is similar although not as strong as caffeine. Theobromine is also obtained in cocoa drinks like hot chocolate. Being high in sugar and stimulants, plus its delicious taste, it's easy to become a chocaholic. The best way to quit the habit is to have one month with NO chocolate. Instead you can eat healthy 'sweets' from health food shops. My favourites are Sunflower bars and Karriba bars. After a month you will have lost the craving for chocolate.

Cola and some other fizzy drinks contain between 5 and 7mg of caffeine which is a quarter of that found in a weak cup of coffee. In addition, these drinks are often high in sugar and colourings and their net stimulant effect can be considerable. Check the ingredients list and stay away from drinks containing caffeine and chemical additives or colourings.

Alcohol is chemically very similar to sugar, and high in calories. It disturbs normal blood sugar balance and appetite. Enough alcohol suppresses appetite which leads to more 'empty' calories from alcohol and less nutritious calories from healthy food. Alcohol also destroys or prevents the absorption of many nutrients including vitamin C, B complex, calcium, magnesium and zinc. Best results are achieved in this diet by being more or less alcohol free. If you drink regularly it is best to have two weeks off alcohol. After that, no more than five glasses of wine or half pints of lager or beer a week is a good target to aim for.

Choosing Alternatives

Bad habits are much easier to break if you have good alternatives to choose from. Nowadays there are many alternatives to tea, coffee, alcohol and chocolate. My favourites are Blackcurrant Bracer, Orange Dazzler and Apple Magic herb teas, Caro Extra, Aqua Libra, and Sunflower bars. Try them out and find out what you like.

Setting Your Target

Set yourself a realistic target for the first month. How to do this is explained fully in the Appendix 'Setting Your Target and Monitoring Your Progress'. This will help you to keep motivated and on track.

Checking Out The Exercises

Rather than fumbling with the exercises on the first day take this week to try them out. Make a nice space in your home to do the exercises. You may wish to get the Fatburner exercise video (see page 158) and do the exercises with the video. Set yourself a time to do the exercises every day, except on your day off. You may wish to double up exercise sessions and have more days off.

With a Little Bit of Help From Your Friends...

Let your friends and your family know what you are doing. Show them this book. Maybe they'll want to join in too! It is good to get a friend doing the diet with you so that you can give each other support. Encourage your family to support you by being tolerant with the new foods you'll be preparing and not tempting you with forbidden foods. When you're invited to dinner let them know about the diet. There are plenty of ways of entertaining on this diet.

You may find it extremely helpful to carry out this diet with the help of a nutrition consultant. See page 158 to find out where your nearest nutritionist is. They will help you to get started and will work out a personalised vitamin programme for you. They will also keep you on track and provide you with moral support and tips on how to deal with any problems you might have.

Be Positive

The world is as you see it, so have a positive outlook. You may have' failed' on diets in the past, however that is no reason to fail again. Most diets don't work in the long-run because they are based on the wrong principles. You can't just will your weight off. The approach must be right. The Fatburner Diet is completely different. You will find it much easier to stick to and will experience many health benefits along the way.

Be positive in what you say and what you think. Replace words like ... "I'll try", "I'll do my best, but..", "I should", "I could" ... with positive statements such as "I am doing the Fatburner Diet", "I am changing my diet", "I am losing weight". Acknowledge youself for what you are achieving. Remember, Rome wasn't built in a day.

The Last Supper

Set yourself a day to start the Fatburner Diet properly. Make sure you have everything you need to get off to a good start. You may want to start at the beginning of the week or the weekend. Celebrate the start of your diet by dining out or preparing your favourite foods the night before. Know that, once you achieve your target, you can enjoy all foods in moderation.

WEEK TWO

Now it's time to get fatburning. Here is a daily schedule to help
you get started. You can swap meals and exercise sessions around
if you prefer.

DAY 1

Breakfast:	Apple Muesli or Get Up & Go, plus supplements
Lunch:	Stuffed Mushrooms
Dinner:	Fish Pie with Watercress Salad followed by Apricot Whisk
Snacks:	Two pieces of fruit
Drinks:	Unlimited water, herb teas, coffee alternatives and diluted juice.
Exercise:	Air-obic session

DAY 2

Breakfast:	Scots Porridge or Get Up & Go, plus supplements
Lunch:	Tofu and Avocado Dip with Crudités
Dinner:	Chickpea Crumble and Green Salad followed by Fruit Salad
Snacks:	Two pieces of fruit
Drinks:	Unlimited water, herb teas, coffee alternatives and diluted juice.
Exercise:	Toning session

DAY 3

Breakfast: Yoghurt Shake or Get Up & Go, plus supplements
Lunch: Rice and Bean Sprout Salad
Dinner: Lentil Lasagne with 4oz lightly steamed Broccoli followed by Raspberry Surprise
Snacks: Two pieces of fruit
Drinks: Unlimited water, herb teas, coffee alternatives and diluted juice.

Exercise: Air-obic session

DAY 4

Breakfast: Pear and Cashew Yoghurt or Get Up & Go, plus supplements
Lunch: Apple and Tuna Salad and 1 slice wholemeal or whole rye bread
Dinner: Tabouli with Tomato and Beansprout Salad followed by Rice Pudding
Snacks: Two pieces of fruit
Drinks: Unlimited water, herb teas, coffee alternatives and diluted juice.

Exercise: Toning session

DAY 5

Breakfast: Scrambled Eggs with 1 slice of wholemeal toast or Get Up & Go, plus supplements
Lunch: Carrot Soup in the Raw
Dinner: Shepherdess Pie, with 4 oz peas followed by Hunza Apricots with Cashew Cream
Snacks: Two pieces of fruit
Drinks: Unlimited water, herb teas, coffee alternatives and diluted juice.

Exercise: Air-obic session and Toning sesssion

DAY 6

Breakfast:	Fruity Oats or Get Up & Go, plus supplements
Lunch:	Cottage Cheese and Alfalfa Sandwich
Dinner:	Sweet and Sour Tofu plus 2oz brown rice followed by Fruit Fool
Snacks:	Two pieces of fruit
Drinks:	Unlimited water, herb teas, coffee alternatives and diluted juice.
Exercise:	None

DAY 7

Breakfast:	Fruit Milkshake or Get Up & Go, plus supplements
Lunch:	Nutty Three Bean Salad
Dinner:	Spaghetti Napolitana followed by Rhubarb and Blackcurrant Pie
Snacks:	Two pieces of fruit
Drinks:	Unlimited water, herb teas, coffee alternatives and diluted juice.
Exercise:	None

WEEK THREE

By now you'll be getting a taste for the Fatburner recipes. Note the ones you like and know that you can exchange lunches or dinners from one day with another day. However, keep your choices varied since some meals are less balanced than others. Week 3 and 4 continue to introduce new and delicious recipes.

DAY 1

Breakfast:	Millet with Fruit and Yoghurt or Get Up & Go, plus supplements
Lunch:	Farmhouse Vegetable Soup
Dinner:	Tamale Pie and Mixed Green Salad followed by Dried Apricot Slice
Snacks:	Two pieces of fruit
Drinks:	Unlimited water, herb teas, coffee alternatives and diluted juice.
Exercise:	Air-obic session and Toning session

DAY 2

Breakfast:	Apricot Nut Shake or Get Up & Go, plus supplements
Lunch:	Potato Salad with 1oz Edam or Gouda or cottage cheese and one banana
Dinner:	Vegetable Pasta followed by Fruit Kebabs
Snacks:	Two pieces of fruit
Drinks:	Unlimited water, herb teas, coffee alternatives and diluted juice.
Exercise:	None

DAY 3

Breakfast: Fruit Cocktail or Get Up & Go, plus supplements
Lunch: Baked Potato, Crudités and Satay Sauce
Dinner: Courgette Quickie on a bed of brown rice with Rainbow Root Salad followed by Apple Crumble
Snacks: Two pieces of fruit
Drinks: Unlimited water, herb teas, coffee alternatives and diluted juice.

Exercise: Air-obic session and Toning session

DAY 4

Breakfast: Kedgeree or Get Up & Go, plus supplements
Lunch: Raw Carrot Soup
Dinner: Chestnut Hotpot with Spinach and Bean Salad followed by Fruit Salad
Snacks: Two pieces of fruit
Drinks: Unlimited water, herb teas, coffee alternatives and diluted juice.

Exercise: None

DAY 5

Breakfast: Muesli with Dried Fruits or Get Up & Go, plus supplements
Lunch: Mexican Bean Dip and Crudites
Dinner: Baked Nut Burgers with Beansprout and Rice Salad followed by Baked Bananas
Snacks: Two pieces of fruit
Drinks: Unlimited water, herb teas, coffee alternatives and diluted juice.

Exercise: Air-obic session and Toning session

DAY 6

Breakfast: Wholewheat or Rye Toast - 2 slices with a little butter and sugar free jam or Get Up & Go, plus supplements
Lunch: Hummus and Crudites
Dinner: Fish Pie with Watercress Salad followed by Apricot Whisk
Snacks: Two pieces of fruit
Drinks: Unlimited water, herb teas, coffee alternatives and diluted juice.

Exercise: None

DAY 7

Breakfast: Banana Breakfast or Get Up & Go, plus supplements
Lunch: Avocado and Orange Salad
Dinner: Vegetable and Nut Flan plus 4oz peas followed by Baked Date and Apple
Snacks: Two pieces of fruit
Drinks: Unlimited water, herb teas, coffee alternatives and diluted juice.

Exercise: None

WEEK FOUR

DAY 1

Breakfast: Scots Porridge or Get Up & Go, plus supplements
Lunch: Lentil Soup and Coleslaw
Dinner: Chicken Salad followed by Rice Pudding
Snacks: Two pieces of fruit
Drinks: Unlimited water, herb teas, coffee alternatives and diluted juice.

Exercise: Air-obic session and Toning session

DAY 2

Breakfast: Fruit Cocktail or Get Up & Go, plus supplements
Lunch: Nutty Three Bean Salad
Dinner: Cheese and Leek Macaroni with Green Salad followed by Fruit Fool
Snacks: Two pieces of fruit
Drinks: Unlimited water, herb teas, coffee alternatives and diluted juice.

Exercise: None

DAY 3

Breakfast: Pear and Cashew Yoghurt or Get Up & Go, plus supplements
Lunch: Butterbean and Sweetcorn Soup
Dinner: Mushroom Pilaf with Tomato and Beansprout Salad followed by Raspberry Surprise
Snacks: Two pieces of fruit
Drinks: Unlimited water, herb teas, coffee alternatives and diluted juice.

Exercise: Air-obic session and Toning session

DAY 4

Breakfast: Banana Muesli or Get Up & Go, plus supplements
Lunch: Hummus and Cheddar Corn Salad
Dinner: Spicy Almond Couscous and Watercress Salad
followed by Rhubarb and Blackcurrant Pie
Snacks: Two pieces of fruit
Drinks: Unlimited water, herb teas, coffee alternatives
and diluted juice.

Exercise: None

DAY 5

Breakfast: Kedgeree or Get Up & Go, plus supplements
Lunch: California Gold
Dinner: Sweet Potato and Pineapple Bake with Green
Salad followed by Raspberry Sorbet
Snacks: Two pieces of fruit
Drinks: Unlimited water, herb teas, coffee alternatives
and diluted juice.

Exercise: Air-obic session and Toning session

DAY 6

Breakfast: Fruity Oats or Get Up & Go, plus supplements
Lunch: Tofu and Avocado Dip with Crudites
Dinner: Spaghetti Napolitana and Watercress Salad
followed by Dried Apricot Slice
Snacks: Two pieces of fruit
Drinks: Unlimited water, herb teas, coffee alternatives
and diluted juice.

Exercise: None

DAY 7

Breakfast: Apricot Nut Shake or Get Up & Go, plus supplements
Lunch: Potato Salad with 4oz grapes and a banana
Dinner: Rice and Bean Casserole with 4oz lightly steamed kale followed by Apple Crumble
Snacks: Two pieces of fruit
Drinks: Unlimited water, herb teas, coffee alternatives and diluted juice.

Exercise: Air-obic session

Maximum Weight Loss

If you have a lot of weight to lose and would be happy eating less here are three ways to speed up your weight loss:

DIET - Either have one day a week eating up to 3 pounds of fresh fruit only, or substitute three main meals during each week with three pieces of fresh fruit. You can make great Fruit Whizzes by liquidizing watermelon, melon, strawberries, raspberries or blackcurrants and other fruits.

EXERCISE - Do five Air-obic exercise sessions per week.

SUPPLEMENTS - Add Konjac fibre to your supplement programme. This usually comes in 500mg capsules, with the recommended intake being nine capsules a day. Take three capsules, with a large glass of water, three times a day just before meals. See Useful Addresses on page 155 for suppliers.

Breaking The Rules

Very few people stick to diets 100 per cent strictly 100 per cent of the time. No doubt there will be the odd occasion when you break the rules. This is not a disaster. In fact, we recommend you give yourself two meals a month when you can eat what you like. This will help you to deal with special occasions and celebrations.

Enjoy yourself. You can always limit the quantity you eat, or substitute a meal the next day with three pieces of fruit. Obviously, the more you break the rules the slower will be your progress. However, watch out for your addictions. These have a nasty habit of creeping back into your life and are best avoided even on special occasions.

What Results Can I Expect?

According to studies on the Fatburner Diet the average weight loss achieved is between 1 and 1.5lbs a week over a twelve week period. That's over a stone in under three months. It is better not to lose weight faster than this. Weight loss of over 2lbs a week is very unlikely to be fat loss. The body simply cannot burn off fat that fast. Of course, most of us want to lose a stone in a week, despite having taken a year to put it on!

Sometimes, after an initial period of weight loss your weight gets stuck at a particular level. This 'plateau' effect is quite common and is no cause for concern. Keep going with the diet, perhaps adding the Maximum Weight Loss recommendations for a couple of weeks.

Remember, the purpose of this diet is to burn fat, not just to lose weight. As your body becomes leaner and fitter more of you is muscle and less is fat. Since muscle is heavier than fat you may lose more inches than pounds. How you feel and how you look is more important than your weight.

What If The Diet Doesn't Work?

No diet works for everyone for the simple reason that there are many different causes for obesity. Some people find it impossible to stick to a diet (although the Fatburner Diet is very easy in comparison to most). Others don't lose weight despite sticking strictly to diets. This can be because there is some other reason why their metabolism isn't working. In this case it is best to get professional advice from a qualified nutrition consultant who can investigate your particular problem or perhaps give the necessary support and guidance you need. There are details on how to find a nutrition consultant near you on pages 155 and 158.

PART THREE

Fatburning Exercises

FATBURNING EXERCISES

To be a Fatburner all you need to
do is the equivalent of
15 minutes exercise a day, or 30 minutes exercise,
three times a week.

This means:
At least three Air-obic sessions per week
At least three toning sessions per week.

*The Air-obic sessions we recommend are one of the following:
Air-obic walking, Air-obic swimming or the
Fatburner Air-obic Circuit.*

Air-obic sessions involve exercise designed to help your body take in, and use more oxygen. It is the reaction of oxygen with carbohydrate that makes energy. To make a roaring fire you need wood and a good draught. Complex carbohydrate is our wood, oxygen the draught. The body's metabolism lights the fire - and burns the fat.

You may prefer to take your air-obic sessions in the form of an aerobic dance class, jogging, cycling, etc. (These options are explained later, on page 111.) If you are significantly overweight and out of condition, you should acquire a base level of fitness by walking or swimming before embarking on the Fatburner Air-obic Circuit or anything as strenuous as jogging or high impact aerobics.

- Both the air-obic and toning sessions can be done on the same day, but I would recommend alternating days, especially for beginners.
- Look at the days and times in your diary that you are planning to exercise; maybe invite a friend or another member of your family, if this will help you stick to your exercise goals.
- Read all the instructions carefully before you start and remember to perform the warm-up exercises first, before every exercise session, whether air-obic or toning.

Before getting started here are a few tips that will help you to stick to your Fatburner exercise programme.

Getting Started

To lose weight you must be motivated. How badly do you want to lose that unsightly fat that covers your potentially gorgeous body? Picture yourself on the beach in a great bathing suit or a special outfit you would like to wear with the person of your dreams. Can you imagine how wonderful it will be not to have to hide your body?

See yourself the way you would like to be and realize that, with time, you can achieve your goals. Don't be put off by the fact that you have tried before and failed. Try again and really tap into that desire to make it work. Remember, everyone has setbacks, even great athletes—that's only human. But don't give in. You may need to take a break from it from time to time, that's OK. But always think positive. You can achieve your goals.

"I'm too busy" is the excuse given by so many active people. Schedule a regular time for exercise, put it in your diary and do not allow yourself to cancel it, except for an emergency. Choose a time that suits you. Some people prefer the early morning when they are fresh and energetic; it helps them start the day right or they just prefer to get it out of the way. Others prefer to exercise during their lunch break instead of having a heavy lunch.

I find exercising after work helps take my mind off work problems or it can just give me the time to think things through. It also energizes me.

Beginners may find that, at the end of the day, it is too easy to make the excuse of being tired; in fact, after a heavy day's work, you may be tired and your exercise programme will seem a chore. If this is the case, exercise before work or during your lunch break.

Set Realistic Goals

It is important that you set realistic goals. (Setting Your Target and Monitoring Your Progress, on page 150, shows you how.) If you set your targets too high, you can easily feel defeated. Set yourself a challenging but realistic routine that you can accomplish. Start off slowly and gradually build. If you have never exercised before, you may find ten minutes of brisk walking tiring. But if you start with five to ten minutes every day, you will soon see improvements.

It takes about eight weeks of exercising regularly for it to become a habit. So stick with it! Also, don't expect results overnight! Plan to make a long-term commitment of at least six months and expect to lose about one pound per week. The slower you lose weight, the greater the chance you have of keeping it off. *Remember, crash diets and heavy exercise programmes are short-lived.*

Be realistic about your body shape. Take a close look at your body. If you have large hips, is it because you are carrying excess fat, or is it because you have large bones? If you have broad hips because of your bone structure, it may not be realistic to expect your hips to become narrow. If you have short legs and a large torso, all the exercise and dieting in the world will not change that. So learn to love your body structure and work on improving it, so that it looks the very best it can.

To start with make it easy to reach your goals. Then if you are comfortable, push yourself a little further. Be patient. Remember progress is made one step at a time.

Motivation

This is the area that lets so many people down. Find what motivates you, what will make you feel good. Maybe it's a new outfit or a new boyfriend or girlfriend. Get in shape for a holiday, then when you return from the holiday, set yourself another target. Keep your target in mind.

If you easily get bored exercising on your own, work out with a friend. You can then motivate each other. If you can afford it, you may find working out with your own personal trainer really helps you. Join an aerobic or circuit training class, a walking association or jogging club. If at home, watching a video or TV or playing inspiring music can take your mind off your workout and help the time fly by. Vary your workout so that you do not become bored.

Stay With It

Most beginners who have been inactive for a long time give up within the first few weeks. They often lack self-confidence and expect too much too soon. They have set unrealistic goals. Be patient.

- When you start to exercise, your muscles may feel sore. Some soreness is to be expected; this will disappear as your body becomes more accustomed to your programme. Remember to warm up and cool down properly.
- You hate exercise! Often this is the case when you choose too hard an exercise programme that does not suit your personal motives or a skill-related activity that you are having trouble with, such as aerobic dance. The answer is to take it one step at a time. Be patient. Don't feel intimidated. Or, just change to another activity that suits you better.
- You may be impatient to see results from your efforts. Don't give in. It takes at least three months to see improvements.
- You may feel tired from the exertion. Give your body time to adjust to the new routine. You will then start to feel stronger and more energized. Don't let these problems discourage you and don't try to compete with others. Go at your own pace. This programme is for you.

You are 62 Per Cent Water!

Water is your most vital nutrient. During exercise you lose a significant amount through perspiration, and through the breath. It is very important to drink before, during and after exercise. For every hour of vigorous exercise, you need to drink approximately an 8oz glass of water. This is especially important while exercising in high temperatures and humidity levels, such as on holiday.

Finding Your Training Heart Rate Zone

To find your training heart rate zone, you need to subtract your age from 220, then calculate 65% of this amount for the lower end of your training zone and 80% for the upper limit, e.g.,

$$220 - \text{Age} = \underline{\quad} \times .65 = \text{lower limit}$$
$$220 - \text{Age} = \underline{\quad} \times .80 = \text{upper limit}$$

For example, for a 30 year old,

$$220 - 30 = 190 \times .65 = \text{lower limit} = 124 \text{ beats per min.}$$
$$220 - 30 = 190 \times .80 = \text{upper limit} = 152 \text{ beats per min.}$$

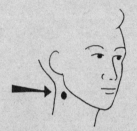

Carotid Pulse

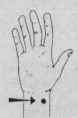

Radial Pulse

To find your pulse rate, you will need a watch with a second hand. There are several points at which the pulse can be felt easily: the neck (the carotid pulse) on either side of the Adam's apple; or the wrist (the radial pulse) on the inside of the wrist just below the thumb.

The carotid pulse is usually the easiest to find for most people. However, if you press too hard on the carotid artery when taking the pulse, it can cause the heart to beat slower. This is not usually the case, but to make sure, try taking the carotid pulse one time and then the radial pulse the next. If there is a difference, determine your pulse by the radial method only. To find your pulse, apply light pressure with your fingers. Do not use your thumb as this has a pulse of its own and will give you an inaccurate count. Normally, for medical examinations your pulse is taken for 60 seconds. But to find your pulse while exercising, stopping for this long would lower your pulse and give you a false reading. So take the pulse

Training Heart Rate Zone Chart (while exercising)

Age	65-80% of maximum heart rate	
	(beats in 1 minute)	(beats in 10 sec.)
20	130-160	22-27
22	129-158	22-26
24	127-157	21-26
26	126-155	21-26
28	125-154	21-26
30	124-152	21-25
32	122-150	20-25
34	121-149	20-25
36	120-147	20-25
38	118-146	20-24
40	117-144	20-24
45	114-140	19-23
50	111-136	19-23
55	107-132	18-22
60	104-128	17-21
65	101-124	17-21
70	98-120	16-20

for only 10 seconds and multiply the result by 6 to give you the number of beats in one minute. This will be your exercising pulse rate.

When you first embark on your Air-obic sessions, you will need to stop briefly every 10-15 minutes to monitor your pulse. After a while you will become familiar with how the correct pulse feels for you.

See the chart above to find your exercise heart rate for your age. The centre column shows how many beats you should have in one minute. Beginners should aim for the lower figure on the left hand side (that is 65% of their maximum heart rate for their age). Then slowly increase to 80% of their maximum heart rate. Do not exceed this higher level.

The column on the far right gives you how many beats you should have in a l0 second pulse count. Beginners should stay at the lower end of their exercise range.

Ready, Steady, Go!

Now you are ready to start your fatburning exercises. Your weekly schedule must include, at least:

1 Three Air-obic sessions, choosing from Air-obic walking, Air-obic swimming and the Fatburner Air-obic Circuit Training.
2 Three Fatburner Body Toning Exercises.
3 Warm up, and cool down exercises before and after each session.

Here are the indications for: Warming up (and cooling down); Air-obic walking; Air-obic swimming: the Fatburner Air-obic Circuit; Fatburner Body Toning Exercises.

Happy Fatburning!

Work out with Bridget with her highly rated Fatburner exercise video. The Fatburner video shows you how to do all theses exercises. Details on how to order are given on page 158.

Warm-Up Exercises

It is important to warm-up your body immediately prior to any exercise session. By gently raising your body temperature and stretching the muscles, ligaments and connective tissue your warm-up will prepare your body for the work to follow and help protect it from injury.

Your warm-up should consist of whole body movements that will raise the muscle and blood temperature, such as brisk walking as a warm-up for your running programme; or a few gentle laps in the pool before you embark on your more vigorous swimming programme; or simply marching on the spot, gentle skipping or dancing to your favourite dance track prior to your Fatburner Body Training Programme.

These body warming movements should then be followed by stretches that will release tension in the muscles. You should not force your body into a stretch position, but progressively ease into a stretch, hold it, then move further into the position if the sensation of stretch subsides. Never force or bounce your limbs into position. Keep your body as relaxed as possible while you are stretching, and breathe gently.

Cool Down

It is equally important to cool down after a bout of heavy exercise. The body must make a number of adaptations during the recovery period before it returns to normal. The muscles that have been pumping the blood back to the heart (e.g., leg muscles when jogging or brisk walking), may build up excess fluid. This may cause stiffness or lightheadedness as the blood pools in the legs. These effects can be prevented by continuing to move the affected muscles in a gentle and rhythmic fashion until the body returns to a near-resting state. Then repeat the warm-up stretches.

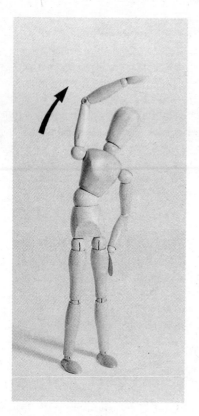 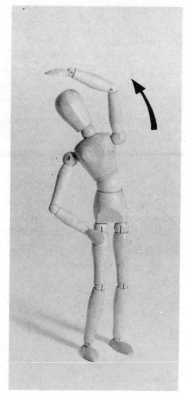

1. Side Stretch

Stand with your feet approximately hip width apart. Bend your knees slightly, keeping your stomach pulled in and buttocks firm. With your left hand on your thigh, stretch your left arm up and over to the right. Return to the centre and then stretch your right arm up and over to the left. Try not to lean forward or backwards. Just stretch up and over to the side.

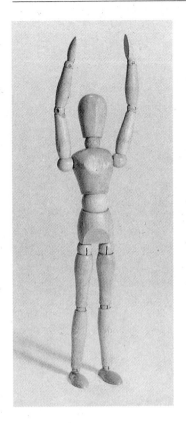 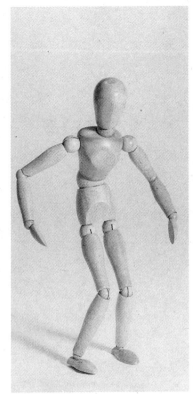

2. Swings

Standing tall with feet hip width apart and facing forward, stretch your arms above your head. Bend your knees and lower your body into a semi-squat position as you swing your arms out behind you. Come back up to standing again as you swing your arms back above your head. Repeat 6-8 times.

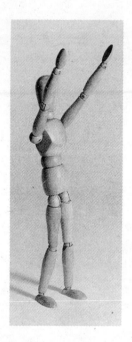 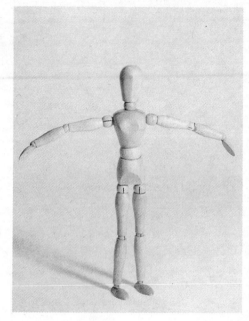

3. Arm Circles

Again standing with your feet hip width apart, circle your arms backwards, sweeping them as close to your ears as possible. Complete the circle by bringing them forwards again. Repeat 6-8 times circling backwards. Then 6-8 times circling towards the front.

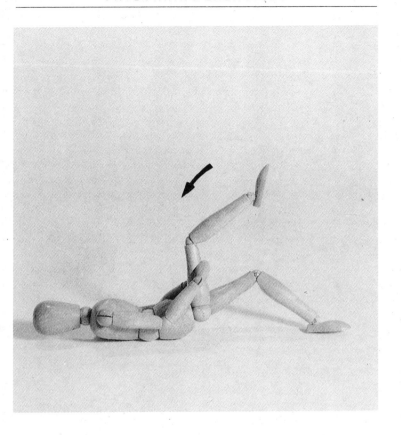

4. Hip and Gluteal Stretch (Buttocks)

Lying flat on your back with your lower back pressing firmly into the ground, bend your right leg and draw the knee in as close as possible to your chest. Hold for 15 seconds, breathing normally throughout. You will feel the stretch around the hip and buttock of the bent leg. Repeat sequence with the other leg.

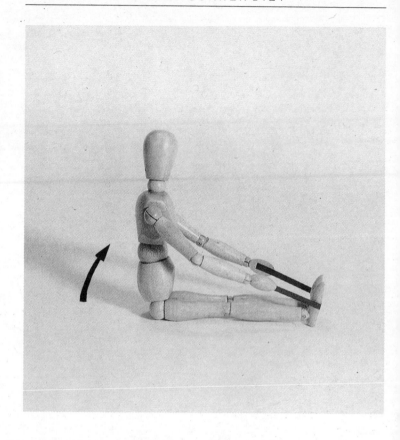

5. Back of Leg Stretch (Hamstrings)

Sit tall with your legs stretched out in front. Keeping your back straight and shoulders relaxed, bend forward like a hinge from the hips (not the waist), and reach towards your feet. Flex your feet by pointing your toes back towards your head. If you cannot reach down far enough to grasp your toes or ankles, loop a strap or towel about your feet. You will feel the stretch in the backs of your legs and you will also feel the muscles of your back working to maintain your long spine position. Hold for 15 seconds, breathing easily throughout.

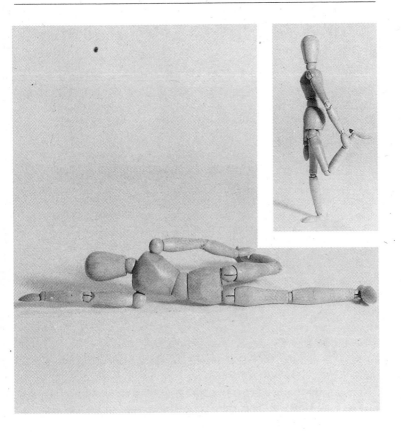

6. Front of Thigh Stretch (Quadriceps)

This exercise can be performed either standing or lying on your side. For standing, you may need to hold onto a chair for support. Reach behind you with your left hand and gently pull the ankle of your left leg towards your left hip until you feel slight discomfort along the front of the thigh. Keep your buttocks tucked under and your spine long. Hold for 15 seconds, then change sides. Again breathe easily throughout.

Air-obic Walking Programme

Walking is a truly excellent form of aerobic exercise for all ages from the novice to the more advanced exerciser. As you become fitter, walking can become more challenging if you add a few hills to your route or use hand weights or carry a backpack or just increase the speed. Walking is accessible and economical, as no special equipment is required—just a comfortable pair of shoes. Compared to jogging, walking is far, far easier on the joints and knees, and can burn about two-thirds as many fat calories.

The latest research studies have shown that people who embark on a moderate walking programme, starting with 30 minutes at 3 miles per hour, lose more weight, keep more weight off, and stay with their exercise routine longer than people who engage in more vigorous exercise such as jogging.

Many fit people think walking is far too easy for them, but once they start are surprised at how hard they can push themselves and what a great workout they can have. Walking can also be mentally very relaxing and can provide a great time to think problems through. In England there are organizations such as the Ramblers Association that will send you information on walks of particular interest or beauty; there are books available on coastal walks or canal walks. So perhaps, on weekends you can involve your whole family in your fitness programme and have a great outing at the same time - or simply use your lunch hour to take a brisk walk in the park.

What To Do

When you first embark on a walking programme focus on the time/duration, not the distance or speed of your walk, for the very out of condition and overweight person 5 minutes a day may be all you can accomplish, then add 2 minutes every few days. If you are starting at this level, try to walk everyday. You will then soon see improvements. After a few weeks, aim to increase your walking time to 20 minutes and be doing 3 sessions per week.

Remember to check your exercise pulse rate regularly, so that you can monitor the intensity at which you are working (so that you are in your fatburning range!) Beginners should exercise at about 65% of their maximum heart rate (see chart on page 69).

Increase your walk time as you feel comfortable. Try to build to about 30 minutes by the end of four weeks. As you become fitter you will have to walk faster to reach your training zone. When you increase your speed, your stride lengthens and so will the distance you cover. A good way to measure your progress is to pick a landmark and compare your time regularly at that location. Remember to warm-up and cool-down with gentle walking and the warm-up stretches. Do not count this as part of your walking time.

Increasing Your Speed

Beginners should aim to complete approximately 1.5 miles in 30 minutes, building to 4 miles in one hour, after approximately 12 weeks.

Remember to start off easy so you can achieve your goals for duration, distance and speed. Then set yourself new goals each week, month or every few months. Keep checking your heart rate to make sure you are fatburning but not over training. (As a rough guide, if you cannot carry on a normal conversation while exercising because you are out of breath, you are overdoing it.) For variety, plan various routes that you could walk in your area. This may be close to your work or home. Even getting off the bus, tube or train one or two stops earlier and walking the remaining part of your journey is a way of building exercise into your life.

Increasing the Intensity

Ways to increase the intensity of your exercise programme:
• Increase the speed that you walk.
• Use arm movements; swing or pump arms as you stride. Add 1 lb wrist weights. This does not build large muscles, but definitely firms the arms (don't use weights on your ankles as this places stress on the knee joints and lower legs).
• Vary your stride—long strides to short fast steps.
• Hike up a hill.
• Climb flights of stairs.
• Walk in sand.
• Wear a back pack (As you get fitter, you could fill it with books!)

Training Chart*

Week	Time minutes per session	Frequency per week	Speed Approx. MPH	Distance Approx. Miles	Calories Approx. Burnt
1&2	20	3	2.0-2.5	0.5-1.0	60-80
3&4	30	3	2.5-3.0	1.0-1.5	100-125
5&6	40	4	3.0-3.5	1.5-2.0	150-200
7&8	45	4	3.0-3.5	2.0-2.5	250-275
9&10	50	5	3.5-4.0	3.0-3.5	275-300
11&12	60	5	3.5-4.0	3.5-4.0	300-350

*This is a rough guide. Do not be disheartened if it takes you 5-6 months to master. Cover 3.5 - 4 miles in one hour.

Facts at 5 MPH:
• Walking a 12-minute mile (5 MPH) can increase fitness levels and burn 53 per cent more calories than a 20-minute mile pace (3 MPH).
• Aerobic walkers (5 MPH) increase cardiorespiratory fitness by an average of 16 per cent, a rate comparable to that achieved by jogging, but without the same risk of injury.

Air-obic Swimming

Swimming is an excellent all-around activity which develops strength, flexibility and stamina. It is relatively cheap and accessible, and as the body weight is supported by the water, there is no strain on the weight-bearing joints, making it an ideal activity for overweight people. In fact, very overweight people who find even walking too strenuous will enjoy the comfort of swimming; as body fat floats in water, they will find they have far greater freedom of movement. This also applies to women in the later months of pregnancy when they want to keep up their fitness programme, but find their bodies feeling too cumbersome to continue their walking or cycling programme. Very pregnant women love the feeling of freedom of movement they experience in the water.

Swimming is a great activity for people new to exercise, pregnant or recovering from an accident or injury. Because you are weightless in water, stress is taken off the joints. Swimming develops cardiovascular fitness and muscular endurance and is great for weight loss.

What To Do

For swimming to be most effective, concentrate on full leg and arm movements. You can increase the resistance by using hand paddles or a float in the water. In tests, the crawl or breast stroke tend to expend more calories than backstroke. If you are a strong swimmer, you will naturally need to swim faster to expend more calories.

Body wt	100 lbs.	120 lbs.	150 lbs.	180 lbs.	200 lbs.
Fast laps	420	530	630	768	846
Slow laps	240	272	320	368	400

Slow swimming refers to approximately 20 yards per minute.
Fast swimming refers to approximately 40 yards per minute.

Figure 9 *Approximate Calories Expended per Hour Swimming*

As with any fitness programme, warm-up prior to your exercise. A few slow laps in the pool should suffice, plus a few stretches to release any tension you may be carrying. An area that can become quite tense from swimming is the neck and shoulders. So before and after your swim, do a few gentle head circles; shoulder and upper back stretches. Drop your chin to your chest and gently roll your head to your right shoulder, then roll the chin back to the chest again and over to the left shoulder (do not do full head circles just half circles to the front). For the shoulders, circle shoulders forwards. Bring them up to your ears, take them back and drop them down again. Repeat four times, then repeat circling your shoulders backwards four times. (Upper Back Stretch - to stretch your upper back) clasp your hands in front of you at chest height and press out to the front as far as possible. You should feel the stretch between your shoulder blades.

As with the walking programme, concentrate first on exercise duration, then increase your speed and distance covered. Remember if you are using swimming solely as your Air-obic workout, you will need to do at least three sessions per week. You may find two slow warm-up lengths in the pool and then five minutes of faster swimming, followed by two slow cool down lengths, is all you can accomplish to begin with. Don't worry, that's fine. Next time you go to the pool try to do seven minutes of fast swimming, then the next time eight or nine minutes, and so on and so forth.

When you have reached 20 minutes of exercise (this does not include your warm-up and cool down laps or your stretches), start to increase your speed. Try to complete an extra length in the pool in the same time scale as before. You will notice you are a little more breathless. Check your exercise pulse rate to see if you are in your training zone.

To increase your workout time to 25 minutes, when you feel comfortable with your new speed and duration, set yourself a new goal. Gradually build up the speed and duration till you are exercising for at least 40 minutes.

Problems

- Swimming is not quite as convenient as walking, you need to get to the pool and change first unless you are lucky to have one in your own home.
- You need to allow time to shower and change.
- Your hair usually needs washing due to the chemicals often used in the water, which can be a problem for women with long hair.
- During hot weather swimming pools can get very crowded.
- Pools are often closed at certain times in the day for private school classes. Be sure to check on opening times.

Fatburner Air-obic Circuit

The Fatburner Air-obic Circuit is an excellent way to burn those excess calories, as you are increasing your aerobic capacity and toning your muscles at the same time, which in turn, increases your ability to burn fat.

Circuit training was developed back in the late 1950's and has been used for many years in physical education programmes in schools, military training, sports training and rehabilitation. It is growing rapidly in popularity with the general public, as it is fun, easy to follow and can be as challenging as you want to make it. There are many benefits from this form of training, the main being the combination of muscle conditioning and aerobic conditioning in one workout session, which saves a great deal of time. People of different fitness, fatness and ability can work out together. A husband and wife can exercise together in the same programme but at different intensities. Fatburner Air-obic Circuit Training or 'variety' training (variety is the key to taking boredom out of exercise), as it is sometimes called, is a variety of exercises linked together to help improve your cardiovascular system and burn body fat.

What to Do

Run through all the exercises first so you can familiarize yourself with the correct technique and form. You will need a watch with a second hand or, ideally, a stop watch so you can time the length of each exercise.

Remember to warm-up first with some mobility exercises for 3-5 minutes (either gently jog on the spot or maybe play your favourite record and dance to it). Follow this with the Warm-up Stretches.

The duration for each exercise is 45 seconds. Your aim is to repeat the exercise with good technique as many times as possible within the 45 second period before moving on to the next exercise. You will then repeat the following exercises as many times as possible (again paying attention to good technique) in the 45 second period, and so on and so forth, until you have completed all eleven exercises.

For your first few exercise sessions, go at a fairly slow pace and monitor your pulse. This will give you a guide as to how much you need to increase your intensity so that you reach your training zone. Walk around the room for 1 minute to recover, then repeat the whole circuit through a second time. Finish with 2-3 minutes of gentle walking to get your pulse rate back to normal and then repeat the Warm-up Stretches as a cool down.

If you are significantly overweight or are unaccustomed to exercise, stay with just one round of the Fatburning Circuit for a few weeks or until you feel you can accomplish one round comfortably at a reasonable pace. You should be exercising at 65% of your maximum heart rate, not 80%. Then add a second round. Increasing the duration (time) of your exercise session before you increase the intensity.

You need to aim for 3 X 20 minute (excluding the warm-up or cool down) Fatburner Circuit sessions minimum per week.

How to Increase the Intensity

You can make your sessions harder and more challenging by

- Increasing the repetitions that you perform in the 45 second period.
- Repeating the circuit 2 or 3 times through, therefore increasing the duration of your exercise session.
- Moving faster from one exercise to another, therefore allowing no recovery time between exercises.
- Adding resistance to your toning exercises, i.e., by using hand held weights for the bicep curls or rubber exercise tubing (for ordering details see page 158). This is great for toning the muscles more.

How to Decrease the Intensity

To make the sessions a little easier for yourself,

- Add a 15-30 second recovery between each exercise, but make this an active recovery by walking around the room.
- Stick to one round of exercises, not two.
- Do easier versions of some of the exercises, i.e.:
  4 Do wall push ups instead of floor push ups.
  6 Do tricep dips with legs bent and closer to your bottom as opposed to the legs straight out in front.
  7 Step up on to a step (8" high only).
  9 In the burpees, walk your feet out behind instead of jumping them out and in.
  11 March on the spot as opposed to jogging on the spot.

Circuit training can be great fun and is an ideal activity to do with friends, as you tend to motivate each other to keep going. Choose some real funky or inspiring music to play while you exercise; you'll be surprised how quickly the time goes by.

The beauty of the Fatburner Air-obic Circuit is that it can be done in the home or in a hotel if you are away on business or holiday, as no special equipment is needed and very little space. Also if the weather is great, you can do it outdoors in the garden, park or on the beach.

As with any exercise programme, listen to your body. If an exercise hurts, check that you are performing it properly, that your body alignment is correct. Go at a slower pace and monitor how you feel. The pain may just be muscle soreness from using muscles you are unaccustomed to using. As you get stronger and fitter this soreness should subside.

Always do the warm-up and cool down stretches, take a bath and relax. Once a week, why not treat yourself to a steam, sauna or massage? You deserve it!

Remember, you can achieve your exercise and weight loss goals if you take it one step at a time; don't give in. You may lapse once in a while, but don't give up. You can do it.

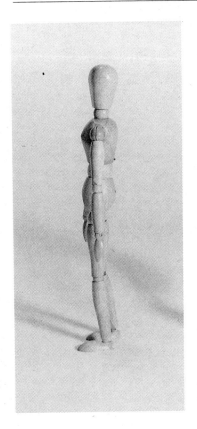 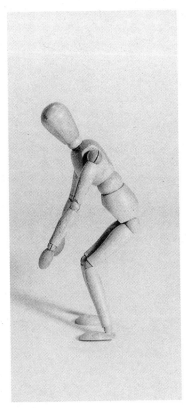

1. Squats

*tones the thighs
and buttocks*

Standing with your feet a little more than hip widths apart, keep your spine long and your stomach pulled firmly in (and facing forward throughout the exercise. Smoothly bend your knees, squatting into a position where your thighs are almost parallel to the floor. (As you squat, make sure your knees run in line with your feet; do not let them roll inwards or out as this puts stress on the knee joints). Gently come up to standing. Repeat the squats as many times as possible in a 45 second period. Move on to Star Jumps.

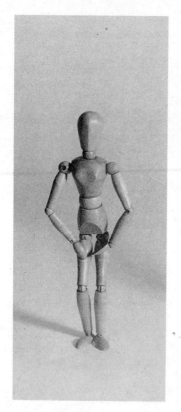 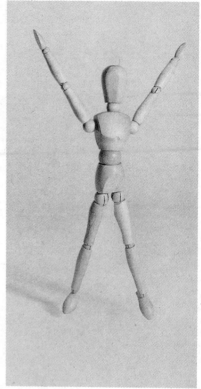

2. Star Jumps   *aerobic*

Standing with your arms by your sides, knees slightly bent and spine long, jump your feet and arms apart as in a star shape. Keep your knees soft as you land, making sure first the balls of the feet and then your heels touch the ground before you jump again. Repeat at your own pace for 45 seconds before moving on to the Backward Lunge.

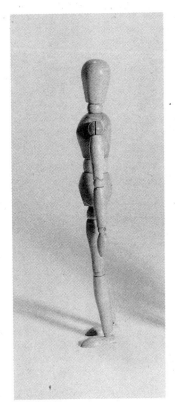 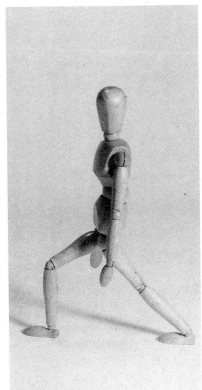

3. Backward Lunge

tones the hips,
buttocks
and thighs

Standing tall with your feet hip width apart, take a large step backwards
with your right foot, lowering your body down into a lunge position.
Your left thigh should be almost parallel to the floor and the knee in line
with your foot. Step your right foot forwards again in line with your left
foot. Then repeat, this time stepping the left foot back. Keeping your
spine long and stomach held firmly in throughout, you can place your
hands on your hips for balance. Repeat, alternating legs for 45 seconds.
Then move on to the Push Ups.

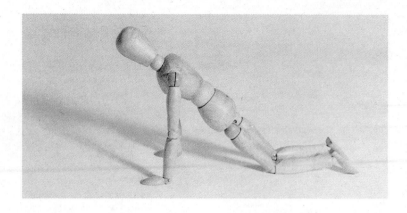

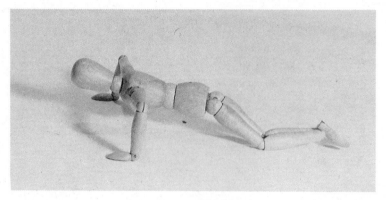

4. Push Ups on Knees   *tones chest,*
front of shoulders
back of upper arms

Adopt an all-fours position with your knees slightly apart. Place your hands parallel a little more than shoulder width apart and fingers pointing forwards. Move your knees backwards until your body is in a straight line from knees to shoulder. Pull your stomach in and firm your buttocks. Slowly bend your arms, lowering your chest so it almost touches the floor. Straighten your arms again and repeat for 45 seconds. Breathe in as you lower and out as you lift. You can make the exercise more or less difficult by moving your knees backwards or forwards. Move on to Single Leg Sprints.

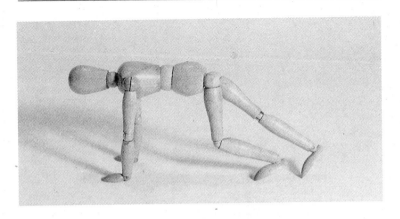

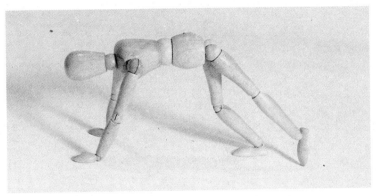

5. Single Leg Sprints   *aerobic*

Support yourself on your hands and feet as though you are going to do a full press up. Your hands should be in line with your shoulders and the spine long. Bring one leg forward toward your chest, keeping the other leg straight. Then smoothly draw the other leg forward as you forcefully extend the bent leg back. Repeat this movement at a steady pace for 45 seconds (if you start to feel light-headed, stop and rest for a few seconds, then continue on to the Tricep Dips).

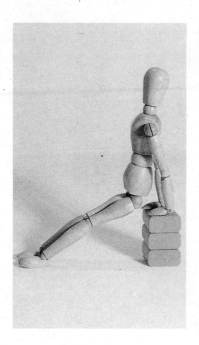 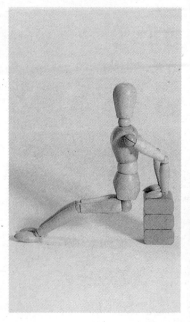

6. Tricep Dips

tones the back of the upper arms and shoulders

Using a chair or bench for support, place your hands approximately hip width apart, fingers pointing towards your bottom and legs stretched out in front (to make this exercise easier, bend your knees and place your feet flat on the floor). Slowly bend your elbows and lower your bottom down towards the floor. Just before your bottom touches the floor, straighten your arms and return to the starting position. Repeat for 45 seconds. Then move onto the Step Ups.

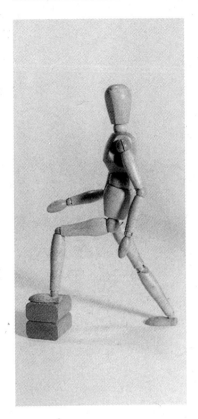 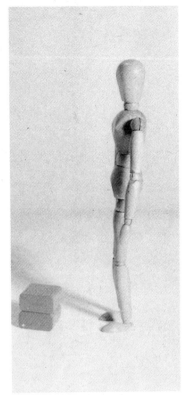

7. Step Ups

*aerobic and tones the
hips, thighs and bottom*

Use either a bench (no more than 12" high) or two steps on your stairs. Stand tall, shoulders relaxed, stomach held firmly in, feet hip width apart. With your right foot, step up onto the bench/step, making sure the full foot is in contact with the step. Do not let the heel drop off behind. Bring the other foot up beside it, then step down with your right foot. Repeat for 20 seconds, stepping up with your right leg leading, then change and step up for 20 seconds with your left leg leading. Move on to Bicep Curls.

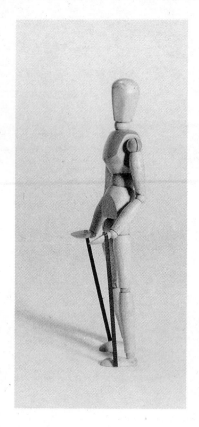 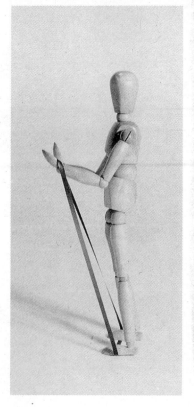

8. Bicep curls

tones the front of your upper arms

For this exercise you can use either hard weights or cans of beans or rubber tubing anchored under your feet. Stand with your feet hip width apart, spine long, buttocks tucked under and shoulders relaxed. Keeping your elbows by your sides, bend your arm. Curling your hands up to your shoulders, slowly straighten your arms again. Keep the movement smooth and controlled. Do not fling your arms. Repeat for 45 seconds. On to the Burpees now.

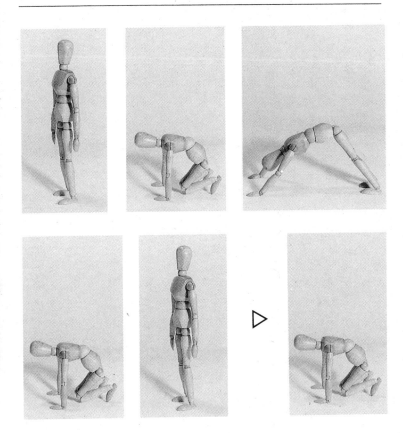

9. Burpees   *aerobic*

A. Standing tall, with your buttocks tucked under and stomach pulled in, squat down as in picture **B**. Place your hands on the floor shoulder width apart and jump your feet out behind, keeping your bottom slightly lifted, as in picture **C**. Jump your feet back in again and come back up to standing. **D** Repeat the sequence again at your own pace for 45 seconds. Progress to Arm Raises.

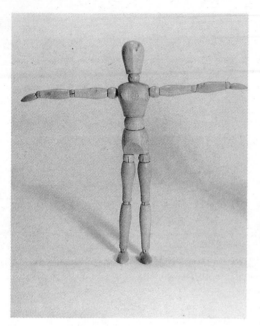 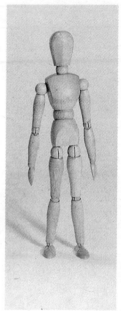

10. Arm raises   *tones shoulders*

Standing with your feet hip width apart, spine long, buttocks tucked under, stomach held firmly in and your shoulders relaxed, slowly raise your arms out to the side and lower. Do not fling your arms; the movements should be smooth and controlled. To make this exercise harder, you can hold 1lb weights in your hands.
Finish with Jogging in Place.

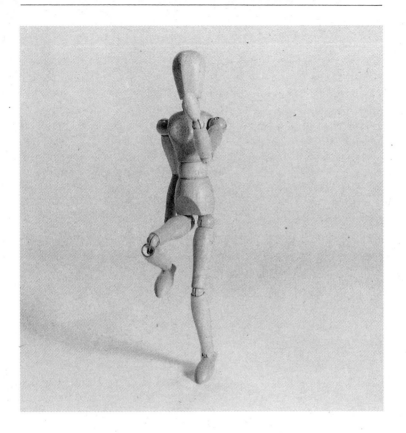

11. Jog in Place   *aerobic*

Gently jog in place, landing first on the ball of your foot and then allowing your heel to contact the floor before springing off with the ball of your feet. You can make this exercise harder by pumping more with your arms and lifting your knees higher. Jog in place for 45 seconds.

Fatburner Body Toning

To remove fat deposits, you have to do large muscle group activities, as in the FatBurner Air-obic Circuit or jogging for example. These will improve overall body leanness. There is no such thing as spot reducing fat, although you can strengthen underlying muscle so that a specific area becomes firmer and tighter.

Every week do three rounds of the following exercises. Do not hold your breath while exercising. Breathe normally throughout; holding your breath can elevate your blood pressure and stress the heart.

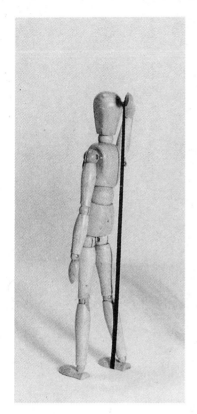 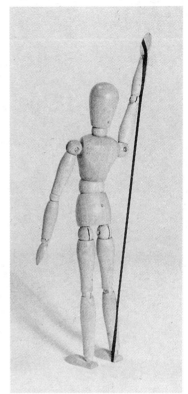

1. Tricep Extensions   *tones back of upper arms*

This exercise can be performed with either a small hand held weight, rubber tubing or band or even with a can of beans as a weight.

Stand tall, knees slightly bent, buttocks tucked under. If using rubber tubing as resistance, tread on it firmly with your right foot, then bend your right arm and grip the other end of the tube behind your head. Point your elbow up to the ceiling. Slowly straighten your arm so that your hand is pointing to the ceiling ; now gently, with control, bend your arm again. Repeat 20-30 times. Change sides and repeat, straightening your left arm, with the tubing anchored under the left foot. If using a hand weight the arm movement will be the same.

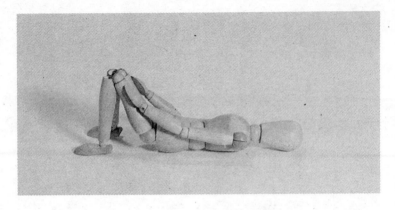

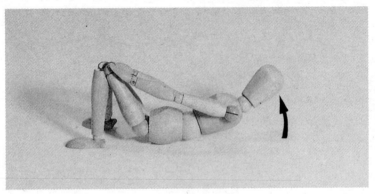

2. Abdominal Curl Ups *tones abdomen*

Lie on your back with knees bent and feet hip width apart. With your hands placed on your thighs, press your lower back into the floor at all times; slowly curl your head and shoulders off the floor reaching your hands towards your knees. Slowly curl down and repeat 20-30 times. Try not to relax in between curls. Keep your breathing relaxed, exhaling as you come up and inhaling as you go down. If you feel a strain on your neck, use one hand to support your head and neck.

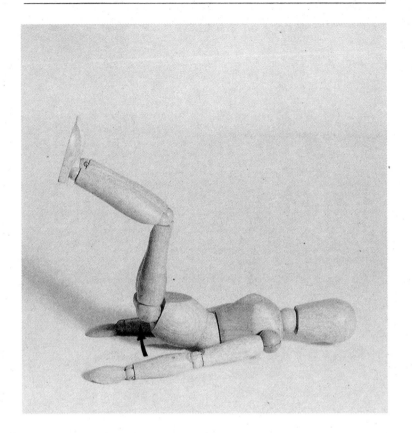

3. Pelvic Lifts   *tones abdomen*

Lie on the floor with your back pressing into the floor, arms loosely at your sides. With your legs at a right angle, your thighs should be vertical and knees over your hips, not your chest. Pull your stomach in and contract your abdominal muscles as you lift your bottom slightly off the floor. (Do not press down into the floor with your hands.) Repeat 20-30 times, exhaling as you lift your buttocks.

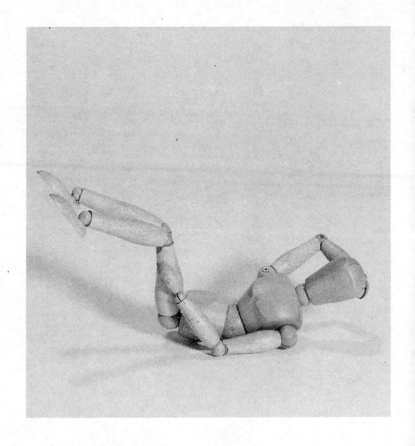

4. Crunch & Twist   *tones waist and abdomen*

Lie on your back with legs bent at a right angle. Using your right hand to
support your neck and your left hand grasping your left thigh to assist in
lifting your torso up higher, slowly release and lower your right shoulder
back down to the floor. Repeat 15 times, twisting the right shoulder across
to the left knee; then change and twist the left shoulder across to the right
knee. Exhale as you come up and inhale as you lower.

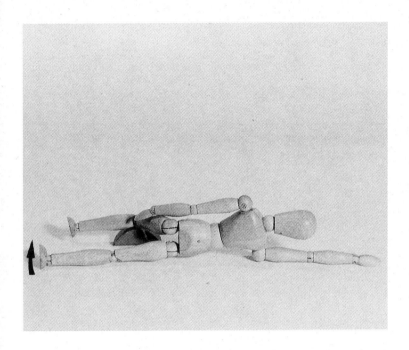

5. Inner Thigh Toner   *tones thighs*

Lying on your right side resting your head on your arm, bend your left leg and rest your knee on the floor or on a cushion for support. Keeping your right leg straight, slowly raise it off the floor as high as possible, then gently with control lower it to within a few inches off the floor; then raise again. Repeat lifting the leg 20-30 times, not allowing it to relax in between lifts. Change sides and repeat with the left leg.

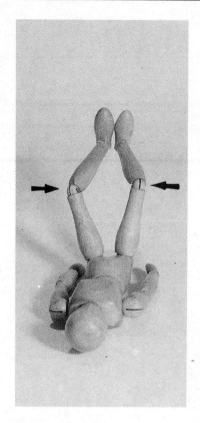 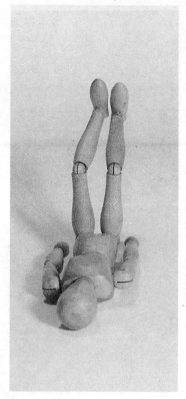

6. Butterfly   *shapes inner thigh*

Lying on the floor, with your spine long and lower back in contact with the floor, bend your knees at a right angle and press the inside edges of your feet together with knees turned out. Slowly press your knees together, then open again. Imagine you are squeezing a large beach ball between your thighs as you press your knees in towards each other. Repeat 20-30 times.

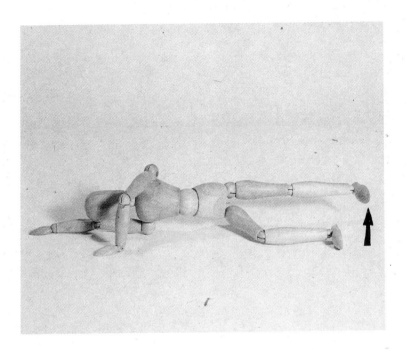

7. Straight Leg Side Lift *tones hips and outer thighs*

Lying on your left side, rest your head on your arm and bend your left leg slightly for balance. Keep both hips facing directly forwards. Extend your right leg out straight to the side so that your right shoulder, hip, knee and ankle are in line. Leaning forwards slightly onto your right arm will help with your alignment. With control lift and lower your straight leg with the emphasis on lengthening it as far as possible as you lift it. Do not lower the leg completely to the ground in between lifts. Repeat 20-30 times, then move onto the next outer thigh exercise (Bent Leg Side Lift). Do all three outer thigh exercises in sequence, not changing sides yet.

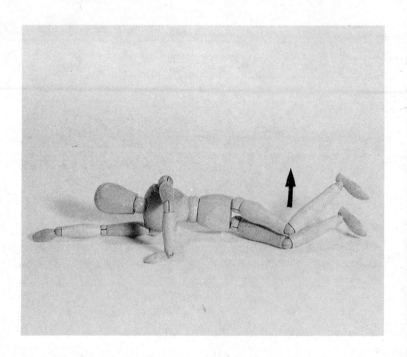

8. Bent Leg Side Lift *tones outer thigh and side of buttocks*

Still in the same position as the previous exercise, bend your right knee and raise the right foot slightly towards the ceiling, leaning a little further forwards onto your right hand. Keeping the right leg bent at this angle, slowly lift and lower the leg. Do not relax in between lifts. Repeat 20-30 times, then move onto the final hip and thigh exercise before changing sides.

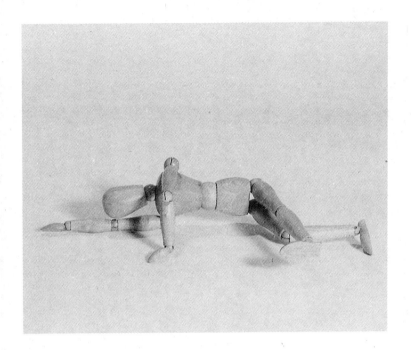

9. Leg Lift to Front   *tones buttocks*

Again with the same side lying position, extend the right leg in front at
a 45 degree angle. It is very important that the right hip does not roll
backwards; if anything, it should be rolled slightly to the front. Flex your
right foot and as you reach out through your heel, gently lift and lower
your leg approximately two feet. Repeat 20-30 times. Then change sides
and repeat the last three thigh exercises lying on your right side and using
your left leg.

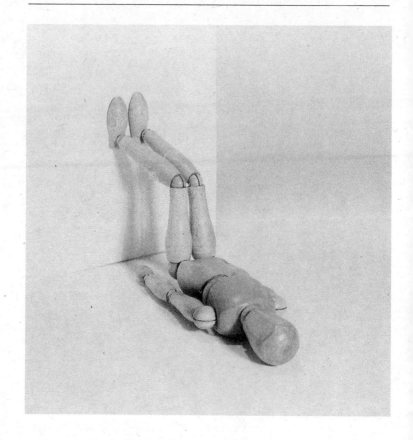

10. Buttock Lifts   *tones buttocks*

Lying on your back with your spine long and stomach held firmly in, bend your knees at a right angle and place your feet on the wall. Squeeze your buttocks tight as you lift your bottom slightly off the floor. Make sure the small of your back stays in contact with the floor. Gently squeeze and release your buttocks, but do not relax your bottom down to the floor between contractions. Repeat the squeezes 20-30 times.

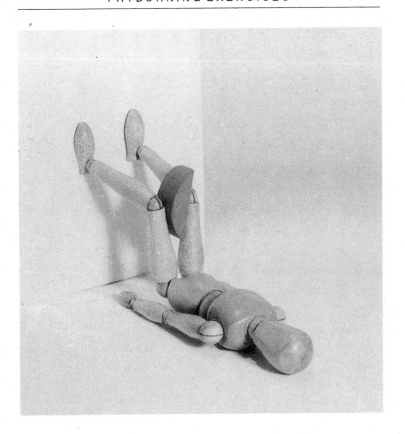

11. Buttock Tucks with Cushion *tones buttocks and inner thighs*

Still in the same position as the previous exercise, grip a cushion or ball between your thighs. Press your knees together and raise your hips slightly off the floor. Repeat squeezing and releasing 20-30 times.

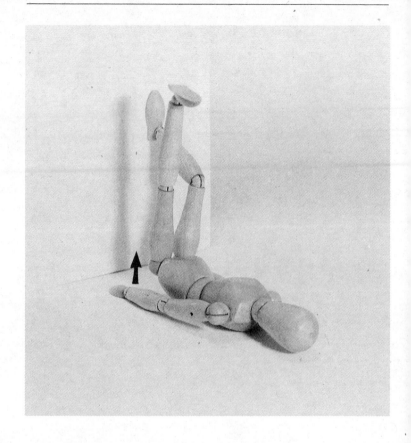

12. Buttock Squeeze with Leg Extended

tones buttocks and back of thighs

Still assuming the same position with legs bent, small of your back pressing into the floor, spine long, and arms loosely at your sides, extend your left leg to the ceiling directly about your hip. Squeeze your buttocks together again and lift your hips slightly off the floor. Repeat 20 little buttock squeezes with lifts, making sure the small of your back does not come off the floor. Repeat, but now with your right leg extended to the ceiling. Finish by hugging your knees into your chest and relax.

Other Exercise Options

To add variety to your exercise programme you may want to swap some sessions for other forms of exercise. Here are some you may like to try, with their advantages and disadvantages.

Running

Running is the quickest method of attaining the minimum level of aerobic fitness. Running is accessible and economical - the only necessity being a pair of good running shoes. On the minus side, running can become boring if done alone. If running in a city, pollution is a problem. Also, running has no effect on exercising the upper body, and injuries are very common, especially when running on hard surfaces. The impact of each jogging step is three times your body weight. Knee injuries are the most common, followed by injuries to the lower legs and feet. These potential problems can be overcome by investing in top quality shoes and avoiding hard surfaces; try to run on grass or soft surfaces.

Rope Skipping

Skipping is accessible, very economical and a very effective method of attaining aerobic fitness. Skipping works the arms to a certain degree and develops co-ordination. Skipping is not recommended if you are overweight as excess strain can result in knee, ankle, shin or lower back injuries. It also puts stress on the delicate bones of the feet. Skipping for 20 minutes or so continuously also involves a certain amount of skill. Again, cushioned training shoes are recommended to reduce the impact, or skip on a soft floor surface such as grass.

Cycling

Cycling is accessible, relatively economical and a good way to acquire aerobic fitness. Cycling is preferable for overweight people, as there is no strain on the joints. If you find cycling on a stationary bike to be boring, try watching videos or your favourite TV programmes. Getting a rack so that you can read a book or magazine will make your exercise time fly by. If cycling outdoors in a city or built-up area, it is advisable to wear a face mask that filters pollution as levels on our roads are so high.

Tennis

Tennis is essentially an intermittent (stop-start) activity and therefore is not generally called aerobic, as it requires short bursts of energy compared to the steady continuous energy required in running or brisk walking. However, a real novice may get a fairly consistent aerobic workout by the sheer fact that he spends all his time madly chasing the ball around the court. As tennis is a very enjoyable activity, it is probably advisable to get fit to play tennis, rather than use tennis as a means of becoming fit.

Squash/Basketball/Football

As with tennis, there are intermittent sports demanding short bursts of more concentrated activity. Squash, in particular, is too strenuous a game to be used by the overweight person to acquire fitness. With football it depends on the position you play as to how aerobic the activity is. As before, it is advisable to get fit to enjoy these sports rather than use the sport to become fit.

PART FOUR

Fat burning Recipes

PART FOUR
FATBURNING
RECIPES

If you equate healthy food with endless salads and boring bean dishes these recipes will prove an extremely pleasant surprise. Each recipe is balanced according to the principles in this book, to help your metabolism to work properly.

Almost all recipes are sugar-free, using the natural sweetness present in food. They are also high in fibre, so you don't need to add any extra. We've also used foods that are naturally high in vital vitamins and minerals. We recommend you to buy the freshest ingredients, organic if possible, since these tend to contain more nutrients.

As this diet is mainly based on vegetables, fruits, beans, lentils and wholegrains you will find it very economical. You may need to vary the fruits and vegetables depending on what's in season.

A few recipes refer to 'sautéeing'. This is quite different from frying. Use a fraction of butter or olive oil, just to lightly coat the saucepan. Warm the oil and add the ingredients. As soon as they are sizzling, after a couple of minutes, add two tablespoons of water or vegetable stock and cook with the lid on. In this way vegetables can be 'steam-fried' using a fraction of the fat used in frying, and taste delicious.

To follow the Fatburner Diet all you need to do is select a breakfast, lunch, dinner and dessert, for each day. Not all the recipes have exactly the same balance of nutrients so its best to vary your choices, as recommended in Part Two. Some lunches and dinners give quantities for two or four people. So don't forget to divide the quantities accordingly if you're cooking for one!

BREAKFASTS

Breakfast is the most important meal of the day, since your body's sugar level is at its lowest. If you go to work very early, take your breakfast to work and have it in a break.

Get Up & Go

Get Up & Go is a breakfast drink made by blending skimmed milk or soya milk with a banana and a serving of Get Up & Go. Get Up and Go is a nutrient rich powder containing complex carbohydrates, protein derived from quinoa, vitamins, minerals, sesame, sunflower and pumpkin seeds, oatgerm, oatbran and beneficial bacteria. Each serving provides the RDA of every known essential nutrient plus many more as yet without RDAs from essential fatty acids to beneficial bacteria, a third of all the protein you need, plus complex carbohydrate, fibre and very little fat. It contains no sucrose, no additives, no animal products, no milk, no wheat and no yeast.

Each serving, with skimmed milk or soya milk and a banana provides less than 300 calories thus making it ideal as part of a balanced low calorie diet. It is nutritionally superior to any other breakfast choice and is totally suitable for adults and children alike. It is fine to have this for breakfast every day, if you choose. It is my breakfast of choice - an excellent way to start the day if you lead a busy life. It is available, by mail-order, from the Fatburner Club (see page 158).

1 serving Get Up & Go

1/2 pint (300ml) skimmed milk or low-fat soya milk
1 banana
1   Blend milk, banana and Get Up & Go powder.

Apple Muesli

Apple Muesli is one of many mueslis you can make yourself. Experiment with other combinations. Apple muesli tastes best soaked overnight in enough water to cover ingredients. Add milk and yoghurt in the morning.

2 tbsp oatflakes
1 tbsp raisins
1 apple, grated
2 tbsp natural yoghurt
1 tbsp (25g) almonds or ground sesame seeds

1 Serve with skimmed milk or low fat soya milk.

(Serves 1)

Scots Porridge

On a cold winter day nothing can be more warming than porridge. Oats contain special factors that are known to promote a healthy heart and arteries and are full of fibre and complex carbohydrates.

1/3 pint (200 ml) water
1/3 pint (200 ml) skimmed milk
1/2 cup (25 g) porridge oats
1 tsp honey or half a banana

1 Put the water and half the milk in a saucepan and sprinkle in the oats.
2 Bring to the boil and boil for two minutes, stirring all the time.
3 Serve with milk and a little honey or half a banana.

(Serves 1)

Yoghurt Shake

Low fat, live yoghurt is a first class food, unlike its commercial counterpart, in which most bacteria have been destroyed for a longer shelf life. Live yoghurt is packed with good bacteria that have a spring-cleaning effect on your digestive system, as well as being a fine source of protein.

5 oz (125 g) very low fat yoghurt
1 banana or other fruit

1 Combine all the ingredients in a blender. Use any fruit that is in season.

(Serves 1)

Pear and Cashew Yoghurt

Live yoghurt, jazzed up with pear and cashew, is a great way to start the day.

1 pear
5 oz (125 g) very low fat yoghurt
1 tbsp (25g) of cashews or almonds
1 tbsp wheatgerm

1 Chop pear and combine with all other ingredients.

(Serves 1)

Scrambled Egg

While eggs are rather high in fats, as an occasional part of a balanced diet, they are a good source of protein and add variety.

1 free range egg
1 tbsp parsley
1/2 oz (10 g) butter

1 Melt butter in a small saucepan. Add beaten eggs and parsley.

2 Cook slowly, stirring constantly.

3 Serve with wholewheat or whole rye toast.

(Serves 1)

Fruity Oats

This satisfying breakfast is a good source of fibre, as well as essential fatty acids - those fats which are essential to our well being.

1 tbsp oat flakes
1 apple, grated
1 banana, chopped
Juice of one orange
1 dsp (17g) sunflower seeds
Pinch mixed spice

1 Soak oats overnight.

2 Combine with other ingredients.

(Serves 1)

Fruit Milkshake

This is really a hundred different breakfasts depending on the fruit that you use. Try it with peaches and strawberries or banana and fresh dates. As a treat have a mango milkshake.

2oz (50 g) fruit

1 tbsp (25g) ground almonds

1/2 tbsp desiccated coconut

1/4 pint (150 ml) skimmed milk

1 Liquidize fruit, almonds, coconut and some ice.

2 Add milk and liquidize again.

(Serves 1)

Millet with Fruit and Yoghurt

2 oz (50 g) millet

5 oz (125 g) low fat yoghurt

3 oz (75 g) peaches, berries or banana

1 tbsp sesame seeds

1 Soak millet overnight.

2 Simmer millet for 25 minutes.

3 Combine all the ingredients.

(Serves 1)

Apricot Nut Shake

This is a dairy free alternative to milkshakes and provides an instant and sustaining breakfast.

1 cup water

2 oz (50 g) almonds

6 apricots (dried or fresh)

1 tbsp sunflower seeds

1 tbsp wheatgerm

1 If using dried apricots, soak overnight.

2 Blend nuts, seeds and water until smooth. Blend in apricots and wheatgerm.

(Serves 1)

Fruit Cocktail

Use whatever fruits are in season - grated apple and banana, orange and banana, orange and peach or a mix of strawberries, raspberries, red- and black-currants.

1/4 tsp vanilla essence
4 oz (100 g) fruit

1 Liquidize all the ingredients together with some ice.

(Serves 1)

Kedgeree

When cooking brown rice it is important not to overcook it. Apart from the fact that it will be stodgy and unpleasant, overcooking it transforms it from a complex to a simple carbohydrate. The rice should still be in separate grains and not have the appearance of splitting out of its skin.

12 oz (300 g) colouring free smoked haddock
8 oz (200 g) brown rice
1.25 pints (750 ml) water
1 egg
parsley
paprika

1 Bring the water to the boil, add rice and boil for 25 minutes with lid tightly on.
2 Meanwhile steam the haddock in a little water.
3 Combine the flaked haddock and rice.
4 Hard boil the egg, slice and add to the haddock and rice. Garnish with parsley and paprika.

(Serves 4)

Muesli with Dried Fruits

Follow the recipe for Apple Muesli, but replace the apple with a selection of soaked and chopped dried fruits. Add a pinch of mixed spice.

(Serves 1)

Banana Breakfast

Banana and crunchy coconut chips are the best foods to add to yoghurt because the citric acid in fruits like oranges rapidly destroys the beneficial bacteria.

1 banana
5 oz (150 g) very low fat yoghurt
1 tbsp of toasted coconut chips
3 dates

1 Chop banana and combine with all other ingredients.
(Serves 1)

Banana Muesli

Follow the recipe for Apple Muesli, but replace the apple with a chopped banana.
(Serves 1)

LUNCHES

These lunches are all quick and easy to prepare. Many can be made and refrigerated. To save time you may want to make enough for two or three days. Most of these recipes are easy to take to work.

Stuffed Mushrooms

Mushrooms are highly nutritious, containing vitamins, minerals and protein.

10 large button mushrooms
1oz (25 g) ground almonds
3 tbsp yoghurt
2 tbsp parsley
1 stick celery
1 spring onion

1 Clean the mushrooms and remove the stalks.
2 Combine the yoghurt, almonds, parsley and finely chopped celery and spring onion.
3 Use this mixture to fill the mushroom cups.

(Serves 1)

Tofu and Avocado Dip with Crudites

Tofu, a curd made from soya beans, is an excellent source of protein. This delicous dip allows you to crunch away on a variety of raw vegetables.

4 oz (100 g) tofu
1/2 ripe avocado
2 tbsps Quark or other low fat soft cheese
1 clove garlic
1 spring onion
1 tbsp parsley
Pinch paprika
1 tsp tamari or soya sauce
Black pepper

1 Blend all the ingredients until smooth.
2 Serve with a variety of seasonal crudites - carrots, cucumber, tomato, lettuce, celery, fennel, endive, chinese leaves, mushrooms, peppers, cauliflower or broccoli.

(Serves 2)

Rice and Bean Sprout Salad

Bean sprouts, being vegetable in their youth, are incredibly rich in nutrients and high in vitality.

4 oz (100 g) brown rice, cooked
2 tbsp French dressing
4 oz (100 g) bean sprouts
1 carrot, chopped
1 spring onion, finely sliced

1 Pour the dressing over the hot rice and allow it to cool.
2 Combine with the other ingredients.
(Serves 1)

Apple and Tuna Salad

Tuna fish is rich in EFAs and protein.

1 red apple, chopped
1 small tin tuna fish in brine
2 sticks celery, sliced
1/3 iceberg lettuce, sliced
1 handful beansprouts
1 tbsp mayonnaise
2 tbsp natural yoghurt
Black pepper

1 Drain the tuna fish and combine with other salad ingredients.
2 Blend the mayonnaise and yoghurt and mix in to the salad. Season with black pepper.
(Serves 2)

Carrot Soup in the Raw

Ever had a hot, raw soup? This soup is made cold and heated gently, keeping all the vitamin and mineral content intact. It's also full of fibre. Don't overheat it.

1lb (450 g) carrots
2 tbsp (50 g) ground almonds
1/2 pint skimmed milk
1 tsp vegetable stock
1 tsp mixed herbs

1 Place carrots in a food processor and blend to a puree.
2 Add other ingredients and process until mixed.
3 Warm very gently in a pan.
(Serves 4)

Cottage Cheese and Alfalfa Sandwich

Cottage cheese is the lowest fat cheese and contains the minerals high in all milk products. Combined with alfalfa sprouts, it makes a great sandwich mix.

2 oz (50 g) cottage cheese
Large handful alfalfa sprouts
2 slices lightly buttered wholewheat or rye bread
(Serves 1)

Nutty Three Bean Salad

No foods are better than beans for satisfying your appetite and giving stamina.

4 oz (100 g) mixed beans (eg haricots, kidney and flageolet) cooked
A handful of walnuts
Parsley
1 tbsp French dressing
2 oz (50 g) fennel, chopped
2 spring onions, finely sliced

1 Combine all the ingredients.
(Serves 1)

Farmhouse Vegetable Soup

Here's a wonderfully warming and easy to make meal in itself.

1.5lb (700 g) chopped fresh seasonal vegetables, eg potatoes, swede, celeriac, leeks, celery, carrots, broccoli, cabbage.
1 medium onion
2 cloves garlic
1 14oz (450 g) tin tomatoes
1 tbsp olive oil
1 tsp vegetable stock

1 Sauté the onion and garlic in the oil.
2 Add the vegetables, tomatoes, enough water to cover and the vegetable stock.
3 Simmer until vegetables are cooked.

This soup can be liquidized or may be left as it is. Use potatoes in moderation as they thicken the soup.
(Serves 4)

Potato and Chives Salad

Potatoes are a source of complex carbohydrate - as long as you don't overcook them! Eat slightly hard.

2lb (900 g) cold boiled potatoes
1 tbsp chopped chives
2 tbsp low fat mayonnaise
2 tbsp low fat yoghurt
1 spring onion
Black pepper

1 Dice potatoes
2 Combine with other ingredients.

(Serves 4)

Baked Potato, Crudités and Satay Sauce

Potatoes are always unfairly left out of slimming recipes. But do eat the skins since they're full of fibre. When making your own, cook them for as short a time as possible, till they are cooked but crispy inside.

1 baked potato
1 tbsp peanut butter
1 tbsp tahini
1/2 tbsp lemon juice
1 clove garlic
A little vegetable stock

Blend together the sauce ingredients. Serve with the baked potato and a mixture of raw vegetables as crudites.

(Serves 1)

Mexican Bean Dip and Crudités

This spicy red bean dip is a great accompaniment to raw vegetables.

4 oz (100 g) kidney beans, cooked
4 oz (100 g) Quark or other low fat soft cheese
1 tbsp olive oil
1/2 onion, finely chopped
1 clove garlic, crushed
2 tbsp yoghurt
Pinch chilli powder

1 Sauté the onion and garlic gently and add the chilli powder. Cool.
2 Blend all the ingredients, adding more yoghurt if necessary to give a smooth creamy dip. Serve with a mixture of raw vegetable crudités.

(Serves 4)

Hummus

Chick peas, also known as garbanzo beans, have a unique taste which combines well with tahini, a paste of ground sesame seeds. Try sprouting your chick peas first, increasing their vitamin and mineral content.

4 oz (100 g) chick peas, cooked
1 clove garlic, crushed
1 tbsp olive oil
Juice 1 lemon
2 tbsp tahini
Cayenne pepper

1 Place all the ingredients in a food processor and blend until smooth and creamy, adding extra water if necessary.
2 Garnish with a little cayenne pepper.

(Serves 4)

Avocado and Orange Salad

Avocados, although high in fat, are highly nutritious in other respects and are fine eaten infrequently.

1 avocado
1 orange
1 tbsp olive oil
1 tsp Tabasco sauce
Pinch nutmeg

1 Cube the avocado. Peel and slice half the orange.
2 Juice the other half of the orange and mix with the other dressing ingredients.
3 Mix all the ingredients together gently.
(*Serves 2*)

Lentil Soup

Lentils are excellent energy foods and provide good protein as well as plenty of vitamins and minerals. This is an excellent winter dish that only takes 25 minutes to prepare.

8 oz (225 g) brown or green lentils, washed
1.25 pints (750 ml) water
14 oz (400 g) tin tomatoes
1 tsp oregano
2 cloves garlic, crushed
1 tsp vegetable stock
Freshly ground black pepper

1 Simmer lentils until tender in water in a covered pan.
2 Add remaining ingredients and simmer for 5 minutes.
(*Serves 4*)

Carrot Coleslaw

Cabbages are packed with vitamins and minerals. Carrots are high in vitamin A, and onions, high in sulphur containing amino acids, which help to remove toxins from the body.

1 lb (450 g) red or white cabbage
8 oz (225 g) carrots
1 small onion
4 oz (100 g) raisins
2 tbsp low fat mayonnaise
2 tbsp very low fat yoghurt
1 tbsp skimmed milk

1 Finely chop cabbage, carrots and onion.
2 Mix all ingredients. Serve with celery and carrot sticks.
(Serves 4)

Butter Bean and Sweetcorn Soup

This simple soup takes 15 minutes to make.

12 oz (350 g) frozen sweetcorn kernels
1 oz (25 g) butter
1 clove garlic, crushed
1 onion, chopped
2 sticks celery, chopped
4 oz (125 g) butter beans, cooked
1 pinch thyme
1/2 pint (300 ml) skimmed milk
1/2 pint (300 ml) vegetable stock
Black pepper

1 Sauté the onion, celery and garlic.
2 Add remaining ingredients and simmer for 10 minutes.
(Serves 4)

Cheddar Corn Salad with Cashew Dressing

The combination of nuts, cheese and corn increases protein quality as well as tasting delicious.

For the salad:

2 oz (50 g) low fat cheddar cheese, grated

1/2 iceberg lettuce, chopped

1 small green pepper, sliced

2 handfuls alfalfa sprouts

Kernels cut from 2 raw corn on the cobs, or 8 oz (200 g) frozen corn, cooked very slightly

4 oz (100 g) cherry tomato halves to garnish

For the dressing:

1 tbsp ground cashews

1 tbsp low fat natural yoghurt

1 tsp low fat mayonnaise

1 tsp skimmed milk

1 Combine all salad ingredients.

2 Mix together the dressing ingredients in a bowl.

3 Toss the salad in the dressing.

(Serves 4)

California Gold

This dish is excellent for unleashing your artistic talent!

1 apple

1 banana

1 nectarine, or other seasonal fruit

1 kiwi fruit

8 grapes (deseeded)

lemon juice

6 oz (175 g) cottage cheese

alfalfa sprouts

1 Slice fruit and arrange on individual dishes.

2 Sprinkle with lemon juice and top with cottage cheese and alfalfa sprouts.

(Serves 4)

MAIN MEALS

Fish Pie

This is a popular fish recipe. Make sure you ask for colouring-free smoked haddock. Smoked haddock was never bright yellow and the dyes used are not good for you anyway.

13 oz (325 g) combined white fish and colouring-free smoked haddock
1/2 oz (10 g) butter
1 tbsp wholemeal flour
5 fl oz (150 ml) skimmed milk
5 oz (150 g) prawns
4 oz (100 g) mushrooms
1 tsp mixed herbs
Black pepper
1.5lb (700 g) potato (mashed)
2 oz (50 g) low fat Cheddar cheese

1 Steam fish for 15 minutes.
2 Make a white sauce using the butter, flour and milk.
3 Combine fish, sauce, prawns, mushrooms and herbs.
4 Place in an over-proof dish and top with mashed potatoes.
5 Sprinkle with cheese. Bake for 30 minutes at 200C, 400F, gas mark 6.

(Serves 4)

Chickpea Crumble

Chickpeas are an excellent food. They can be bought dry, soaked overnight and cooked. Alternatively, tinned chick peas are already cooked.

Filling:

1 small onion, chopped
1 tbsp olive oil
1/2 red pepper, chopped
2 medium potatoes, diced
1 14oz (400 g) tin tomatoes
1 14 oz (400 g) tin chick peas
Pinch cumin

Crumble:

4 oz (100 g) wholemeal flour
2 oz (50 g) butter
1 oz (25 g) oats
1 tbsp sunflower seeds, toasted

1 Sauté onion, celery, red pepper and potatoes.
2 Add other ingredients, simmer for 20 minutes.
3 Rub butter into flour and mix in oats and sunflower seeds.
4 Place chickpea mixture in an ovenproof dish and top with crumble.
5 Bake at 190C, 375F, gas mark 5.

(Serves 4)

Lentil Lasagne

This vegetarian lasagne uses lentils instead of meat.

1 small onion, chopped
1 clove garlic, crushed
1 tbsp olive oil
1/2 tsp cinnamon
1/2 pint (300 ml) vegetable stock
8 oz lasagne (225 g) (wholemeal or green)
2 oz (50 g) low fat Cheddar cheese, grated

Sauce:

1 oz (25 g) butter
1 tbsp wholemeal flour
1/2 pint (300 ml) skimmed milk

1 Sauté the onion and garlic in the oil. Add the cinnamon, lentils and stock and simmer for 45 minutes.
2 Cook the lasagne in boiling water until tender.
3 Make a white sauce and add in half the cheese.
4 Layer the lentil mixture, pasta and sauce into an ovenproof dish. Sprinkle with remaining cheese.
5 Bake at 220 C, 400 F, gas mark 6 for 45-50 minutes.
(Serves 4)

Tabouli

Tabouli is a traditional vegetarian dish using bulgar, which is cracked wheat. It's an excellent source of carbohydrate. Make sure that you buy fine bulgar rather than coarse.

8 oz (225 g) fine bulgar (cracked wheat)
1 onion, chopped
1 bunch finely chopped parsley
3 tbsp fresh mint
2 tbsp olive oil
6 tbsp lemon juice
1/4 cucumber, diced
Black pepper
Lettuce leaves to serve

1 Soak bulgar for 1 - 2 hours in cold water.
2 Drain bulgar and mix with other ingredients.
3 Serve on lettuce leaves in a bowl.
(Serves 4)

Shepherdess Pie

This vegetarian equivalent of shepherds pie is easy to make.

1 tbsp olive oil
1onion, chopped
1 clove garlic, crushed
14 oz (400 g) tin tomatoes
12 oz (300 g) aduki beans, cooked
1 tbsp parsley, choppped
2 tbsp tamari
1.5lb (700 g) mashed potato
2 oz (50 g) low fat Cheddar cheese, grated

1 Sauté onion and garlic in the oil.
2 Add the tomatoes, parsley, aduki beans and tamari. Simmer gently for 15 minutes.
3 Place bean mixture in an ovenproof dish and top with mashed potatoes and cheese.
4 Bake for 35 minutes and 200C, 400F, gas mark 6.

(Serves 4)

Sweet and Sour Tofu

This Chinese style dish has an unusual taste.

1 tbsp olive oil
1 clove garlic, chopped
1 onion, chopped
1 green pepper, chopped
1 carrot, sliced
4 oz (100 g) tin pineapple chunks (unsweetened)
8 oz (200 g) tofu

Sauce:

2 tsp cornflour
4 tbsp pineapple juice
3 tbsp cider vinegar
1 tbsp brown sugar
2 tsp soya sauce
1 tbsp tomato purée

1 Sauté the vegetables in the oil.
2 Combine the sauce ingredients and add to the vegetables together with the pineapple and tofu. Simmer for three minutes, stirring well.

(Serves 4)

Tamale Pie

This is a Mexican style recipe and is a bean and chilli pot topped with cornbread.

1 tbsp olive oil
1 onion, chopped
1 clove garlic, chopped
Pinch chilli powder
1/2 green pepper, chopped
14 oz (400 g) tin kidney beans
14 oz (400 g) tin tomatoes

Topping:

4 oz (125 g) corn meal
1 tbsp wholemeal flour
2 tsp baking powder
1 egg, beaten
3.5 fl oz (100 ml) skimmed milk
2 oz (50 g) low fat Cheddar cheese, grated

1 Sauté the onion, garlic and pepper with the chilli powder.
2 Add the kidney beans and tomatoes and simmer for 5 minutes.
3 Blend the cornmeal, flour and baking powder and beat in the egg, milk and oil to give a thick batter.
4 Spoon over the bean mixture and sprinkle with cheese.
5 Bake at 220C, 425F, gas mark 7 for about 40 minutes until golden.

(Serves 4)

Vegetable Pasta

This dish can be made with any kind of pasta. However, do pick wholewheat pasta. Health food shops now have buckwheat and corn pasta. Try these for a change.

1 tbsp olive oil
1/2 red pepper, diced
1 stick celery, sliced
1 courgette, sliced
2 oz (50 g) fennel, sliced
1/2 oz (10 g) butter
1 tbsp wholemeal flour
1/2 pint (300 ml) skimmed milk
2 oz (50 g) low fat Cheddar, grated
Black pepper
8 oz (225 g) wholemeal pasta shells

1 Make a sauce with the butter, flour and milk. Add the cheese and black pepper to taste.
2 Lightly sauté the vegetables.
3 Boil the pasta until just cooked.
4 Combine all the ingredients and bake at 190C, 375F, gas mark 5 until light brown and bubbling.

(Serves 4)

Courgette Quickie

This Mediterranean style dish is very popular.

1 oz (25 g) butter
1 large onion
1lb (450 g) courgettes, thinly sliced
4 large tomatoes, sliced
3 cloves garlic, crushed
Black pepper
2 oz (50 g) low fat Cheddar cheese, grated
4 tbsp fresh wholemeal breadcrumbs

1 Sauté the onion.
2 Add the garlic, courgettes and tomatoes and simmer until tender but crisp.
3 Season with freshly ground black pepper.
4 Pour into a flameproof dish and sprinkle with cheese and breadcrumbs and grill quickly under a hot grill.

(Serves 4)

Chestnut Hotpot

Chestnuts are the lowest fat nuts by a long way, so enjoy yourself in chestnut season. Out of season you can use dried chestnuts which simply need soaking overnight (and are much easier to prepare!).

5 oz (150 g) dried chestnuts
1 medium onion, sliced
1 oz (25 g) butter
8 oz (225 g) parsnip
8 oz (225 g) potato
8 oz (225 g) swede
8 oz (225 g) turnip
1/2 pint vegetable stock
Black pepper

1 Soak chestnuts overnight.
2 Sauté the onion in the butter.
3 Slice all the vegetables and add to the pot with the stock, pepper and chestnuts.
4 Simmer very gently until chestnuts are just soft, about 30 - 45 minutes.

(Serves 4)

Baked Nut Burgers

Here is a home-made vegetarian alternative to the hamburger!

1 small onion, chopped
1 tbsp olive oil
4 oz (125 g) mixed nuts, finely chopped
4 oz (125 g) peanuts, finely chopped
1 tbsp peanut butter
5 oz (150 g) wholemeal breadcrumbs
1 tbsp parsley, chopped

1 Sauté the onion in the oil and add in the other ingredients. If necessary add a little water to bind.
2 Shape into burgers and place on a non stick tray.
3 Bake at 200C, 400F, gas mark 6 for 30 minutes. Turn them over after fifteen minutes.

(Serves 4)

Vegetable and Nut Flan

This flan is simple to make and very popular.

8 oz (225 g) wholemeal pastry
1/2 red pepper, chopped
1 courgette, sliced
6 oz (175 g) cauliflower florets
2 sticks celery, diced
2 oz (50 g) roasted (unsalted) peanuts, chopped
2 eggs
1/2 pint (300 ml) skimmed milk
1 oz (50 g) low fat cheddar cheese, grated

1 Line a flan dish with pastry and bake.
2 Steam the vegetables for about 1 minute and place into flan.
3 Beat the eggs and milk together and pour on. Top with cheese.
4 Bake at 180C, 350F, gas mark 4 for about 25 minutes, until golden

(Serves 4)

Chicken Salad

Chicken contains half the fat of other meats.

Cold meat from 1/2 a small roast chicken without the skin
3 eating apples, cubed
3 stick celery, chopped
10 oz (275 g) cold boiled potatoes, cubed
5 tbsp low fat mayonnaise
2 tsp horseradish sauce
5 tbsp skimmed milk
1/3 iceberg lettuce
red pepper to garnish

1 Combine all ingredients , except the pepper and lettuce and pile on to a large plate.
2 Decorate with the iceberg lettuce round the edges, and rings of red pepper on top.

(Serves 4)

Cheese and Leek Macaroni

Here's another pasta variation.

1 oz (25 g) butter
8 oz (225 g) leeks, chopped
2 tbsp wholemeal flour
6 oz (175 g) wholewheat macaroni, cooked
1/2 pint (300 ml) skimmed milk
2 oz (50 g) low-fat Cheddar cheese, grated
2 oz (50g) wholemeal breadcrumbs

1 Sauté the leeks in the butter.
2 Stir in the flour and gradually add the milk to make a sauce.
3 Add the macaroni and half of the cheese.
4 Put the mixture into an ovenproof dish and top with the remaining cheese and breadcrumbs.
5 Bake at 200C, 400F, gas mark 6 for 25 minutes until golden brown.

(Serves 4)

Mushroom Pilaf

Mushrooms can be eaten raw in salads, or cooked as in this delicious pilaf. The secret is to cook them slowly. Adding a little water helps to bring out their juices.

8 oz (225 g) brown rice
1/2 oz butter
I tbsp olive oil
1 large onion, chopped
1 pint (600 ml) hot water
2 oz (50 g) raisins
8 oz (225 g) frozen peas
8 oz (225 g) mushrooms, sliced
1 tsp yeast extract
1 tsp finely chopped root ginger
2 tbsp parsley, chopped

1 Gently heat the oil and butter in a heavy frying pan and fry the rice in it until pale brown. Add onion and cook for a further five minutes.
2 Add water, raisins and mushrooms, cover and simmer until liquid is absorbed and rice just tender. Add more hot water if needed.
3 Stir in yeast extract and ginger.
4 Cook frozen peas, drain and add to rice mixture.
5 Serve garnished with parsley.

(Serves 4)

Spicy Almond Couscous

This is a variation on the traditional Moroccan dish. Couscous is an excellent complex carbohydrate dish.

1 tbsp olive oil
8 oz (225 g) courgettes, sliced
I medium onion, sliced
8 oz (225 g) mushrooms, sliced
2 oz (50 g) raisins
2 oz (50 g) flaked almonds
14oz (400 g) tin tomatoes
I red pepper, chopped
2 carrots, sliced
1/2 tsp chilli powder
8 oz (225 g) couscous
1.5 pints (900 ml) boiling water

1 Sauté onions in oil for two minutes.
2 Add the other vegetables and chilli powder and sauté for a further two minutes
3 Add tomatoes, red pepper, raisins and enough water to cover.
4 Simmer until vegetables are tender but still crisp.
5 Pour the boiling water over the couscous and leave to stand for 15 minutes. Serve the vegetables on a bed of couscous.

(Serves 4)

Sweet Potato and Pineapple Bake

Sweet potatoes are rich in vitamin A and are very delicious. They are easy to find these days in supermarkets. As this dish is rather sweet, serve it with a tasty green salad.

3lb (1.4 kg) sweet potatoes
2 oz butter
Juice of 1 orange
1 8 oz (225 g) tin pineapple (unsweetened)

1 Peel the sweet potatoes, cut into pieces, and simmer in water for 15 minutes.
2 Mash the potato with the butter, orange juice and honey.
3 Stir in half of the pineapple chunks. Place in an ovenproof dish, covering with the remaining pineapple.
4 Bake for about 30 minutes at 180C, 350F, gas mark 4.

(Serves 4)

Spaghetti Napolitana

If you've never tried wholewheat or buckwheat spaghetti this is the recipe to try them with. I prefer buckwheat spaghetti but you have to be a bit careful how you cook it. Bring it to the boil, then add cold water, then bring it back to the boil. Do this twice for best results.

12 oz (300 g) wholewheat or buckwheat spaghetti
2 medium onions, sliced*
2 tbsp olive oil
3 carrots, chopped
8 oz (225 g) mushrooms, chopped
I clove garlic, crushed
1 green pepper, chopped
4 oz (100 g) tomato purée
2 tsp concentrated vegetable stock
1 tsp thyme

1 Sauté the onion in the oil.
2 Add the vegetables and sauté for 5 minutes.
3 Add the vegetable stock, thyme, tomato purée and enough water to just cover. Simmer for 20 minutes.
4 Blend in a food processor.
5 Cook the spaghetti in plenty of boiling water for about 12 minutes. Serve topped with the tomato sauce.

(Serves 4)

Rice and Bean Casserole

Combining rice and beans improves protein quality of this dish.

1 tbsp oil
1 onion, chopped
1 red or green pepper, chopped
2 large tomatoes, chopped
8 oz (225 g) kidney (or other) beans, cooked
Black pepper
6 oz (175 g) brown rice
2 tbsp parsley or coriander, chopped

1 Sauté onion and pepper in oil for about 5 minutes.
2 Add tomatoes, rice, black pepper and beans and enough water to just cover.
3 Simmer until water is absorbed and the rice is cooked.
4 Stir in the parsley or coriander and serve.
(Serves 4)

SALADS

Watercress Salad

Watercress is rich in iron and vitamin A and is delicious in salad.

1/2 bunch watercress
1/3 iceberg lettuce, sliced
1/2 cucumber, sliced
1 green pepper, chopped
3 handfuls alfalfa sprouts

1 Combine all the ingredients and toss with 1 tbsp French dressing
(Serves 4)

Green Salad

This simple green salad is a good accompaniment to any meal.

1/3 Cos or other lettuce, chopped
1/4 bulb of fennel, sliced
2 oz (50 g) broccoli tops, chopped
1/4 cucumber, chopped
2 sticks celery, sliced

1 Combine all the ingredients and toss with 1 tbsp French dressing.
(Serve 4)

141

Tomato and Beansprout Salad

Beansprouts are highly nutritious and can either be bought or sprouted at home.

2 beefsteak tomatoes
Beansprouts
2 spring onions

1 Slice tomatoes and mix with beansprouts. Add 1 tbsp French dressing.

(*Serves 4*)

Spinach and Bean Salad

Spinach is an underestimated salad food, but care must be taken in preparing the spinach leaves.

1 lb (450 g) fresh spinach
3 tbsp minced onion
14 oz (350 g) tin kidney beans

For the dressing:
1/2 tbsp olive oil
1 1/2 tbsp lemon juice
1/2 tsp bouillion powder

1 Strip the spinach leaves from the stalk and soak in a tub of cold water.
2 Lift leaves and rinse under running water.
3 Drain and pat dry.
4 Chop the leaves and toss with the onions and half the beans.
5 Arrange the rest of the beans on top.
6 Mix the dressing ingredients together and pour over the salad.

(*Serves 4*)

Rainbow Root Salad

This colourful combination of carrots, parsnips and beetroots is more filling than you think. Go easy on the beetroot and parsnips as their strong tastes can overpower the carrots.

3 medium carrots, grated
1 small parsnip, grated
1 medium beetroot, grated
parsley, finely chopped

1 Combine three root vegetables
2 Mix with island dressing

(*Serves 4*)

SALAD DRESSINGS

French Dressing

This standard french dressing can be jazzed up by adding fresh and dried herbs. Sesame and sunflower oil contain essential fats (EFA's). Use as little dressing as possible on salads.

4 tbsp cold-pressed sesame or sunflower oil
2 tbsp cider vinegar (or balsamic vinegar)
1 tsp French mustard
1 clove garlic, crushed

1 Put all the ingredients in a screw-top jar and shake vigourously. Any extra dressing can be stored in a bottle in the fridge.

Island Dressing

1 small carrot
1 small tomato
1 tbsp tofu
1 tsp mayonnaise
1 tsp ground almonds
1/2 tsp Vecon (vegetable stock)
1 tbsp skimmed milk
nutmeg, grated

1 To make dressing, liquidize carrot and tomato, add in rest of ingredients including nutmeg to taste and mix thoroughly.

DESSERTS

Apricot Whisk

This dessert tastes even better than it looks. Using dried apricots, rich in micronutrients, it can be made all year round.

8 oz (225 g) apricots
1/4 tsp natural vanilla essence
8 fl oz (225 ml) low fat natural yoghurt
8 oz (225 g) Quark or low fat curd cheese
2 egg whites

1 Stew apricots until soft.
2 Blend in a processor, adding the vanilla essence, yoghurt and curd cheese.
3 Whisk egg whites stiffly and fold into apricot mixture.
4 Chill before serving.

(Serves 4)

Fresh Fruit Salad

Adding one or two interesting fruits improves a fruit salad enormously, for example mango, kiwi, fresh lychee, strawberries, fresh dates or melon.

2lb (900 g) mixed fruits
2 oz (50 g) dried apricots

1 Cut fruit into cubes.
2 Stew apricots and liquidize, adding enough water to make a pourable sauce.
3 Pour cooled sauce over fruit.

(Serves 4)

Raspberry Suprise

This fruit fool is also delicous made with strawberries or blackcurrants.

8 oz (225g) raspberries (fresh or frozen and thawed)
4 oz (100 g) fromage frais
1 tsp honey

1 Pile the raspberries into a serving dish. Serve with the fromage frais and add honey to taste.

(Serves 2)

Rice Pudding

This good old-fashioned recipe uses brown rice instead of white rice for more fibre and taste.

4 oz (100 g) brown rice
2 oz (50 g) raisins
1.5 pints (600 ml) skimmed milk
Grated nutmeg
1 tsp honey

1 Put rice, raisins, milk and honey in an ovenproof dish.
2 Stir until the honey is completely dissolved
3 Sprinkle liberally with grated nutmeg.
4 Bake at 150C, 300F, gas mark 2 for two hours.

(Serves 4)

Hunza Apricots with Cashew Cream

The Hunzas often live to over 100, perhaps by eating apricots, high in vitamin A!

8 oz (225 g) Hunza apricots
2 oz (50 g) whole hazelnuts
6 oz (175 g) cashew nuts

1 Soak apricots in boiling water.
2 When soft remove stones and replace with a whole hazelnut.
3 Grind the cashews in a blender until fine. Slowly trickle in water to give a cream-like consistency.
4 Serve apricots with cashew cream arranged in a sundae glass.

(Serves 4)

Fruit Fool

This can be made from most fruits. Pick them in season and freeze to enjoy all year round.

8 oz (225 g) gooseberries or cooking apples
2 oz (50 g) sultanas
1 dsp honey, to taste
1/2 oz (10 g) butter
1/2 pint (250 ml) low fat yoghurt

1 Cook the fruit and sultanas until softened and stir in the butter.
2 Allow fruit to cool and blend in a processor with yoghurt and honey to taste.

(Serves 4)

Rhubarb and Blackcurrant Pie

If you like rhubarb you'll love the combination of rhubarb and blackcurrants in this pie. You can use any seasonal fruits.

1lb (450 g) rhubarb
8 oz (225 g) blackcurrants
1/2 tsp ground ginger
8 oz (225 g) Quark or low fat curd cheese
1/4 pint (150 ml) skimmed milk
I tbsp honey
2 tbsp ground almonds

1 Stew rhubarb and blackcurrants until soft in a small amount of water.
2 Mix in ginger and put in ovenproof dish.
3 Mix curd cheese, milk and honey together thoroughly.
4 Cover fruit with curd cheese mixture.
5 Sprinkle with almonds and lightly toast under a hot grill.
(Serves 4)

Dried Apricot Slice

A highly delicious treat.

6 oz (175 g) dried apricots, soaked
2 oz (50 g) sultanas
3 oz (75 g) dessicated coconut
4 tbsp apple juice

1 Liquidize the apricots, sultanas and half of the coconut.
2 Press firmly into a dish containing a layer of coconut, and sprinkle the top with more coconut,
3 Chill and serve in wedges.
(Serves 4)

Fruit Kebabs

A colourful combination.

1 green apple
1 red apple
2 bananas
Lemon juice
2 oranges
12 black grapes

1 Cube the apples and banana and coat with a little lemon juice to prevent them from going brown.
2 Peel the oranges, removing all the pith, and cut into chunks. Halve the grapes and remove the pips.
3 Put the fruit onto skewers and grill under a high grill or on a barbecue.

(Serves 4)

Apple Crumble

A traditional and filling British dessert.

1lb (450 g) cooking apples
2 cloves
3 tbsp water
3 oz (75 g) butter
2 oz wholewheat flour
2 oz (50 g) muscovado or demerara sugar
4 oz (100 g) oats
1/2 tsp mixed spice

1 Core and slice the apples and lightly cook them with the cloves and water.
2 Rub the butter into the flour and mix in the spice, sugar and oats.
3 Put a layer of the crumble mixture on top of the apples and bake at 190C, 375F, gas mark 5 for about 20 minutes until golden.

(Serves 4)

Baked Bananas

A delicious treat that everyone enjoys.

4 ripe bananas
1 oz (25 g) demerara sugar
2 tbsp water
Lemon juice
Pinch mixed spice

1 Place bananas in a fireproof dish, sprinkle with sugar, spice and lemon juice and add the water.
2 Bake at 180C, 375F, gas mark 5 until brown, basting the bananas occasionally.

(Serves 4)

Baked Date and Apple

The natural sugar in dates helps to sweeten the most sour of cooking apples.

4 oz (100 g) dates
4 large cooking apples
1 tsp cinnamon
1 tbsp honey

1 Chop dates roughly and core apples.
2 Stuff apple centres with dates and place in an ovenproof dish.
3 Sprinkle with cinnamon, and honey if you need it.
4 Pour water over apples to a depth of 1 inch in the bottom of the dish.
5 Bake at 200C, 400F, gas mark 6 for about 45 minutes until soft.

(Serves 4)

Raspberry Sorbet

There are many variations to this theme, which allow you to pick fruit in season, freeze it and use it whenever you want. Just think, raspberries and strawberries all year round!

1lb (450 g) frozen raspberries
2 bananas, chopped into 1/2 inch lengths

1 Freeze the bananas.
2 Remove bananas and raspberries from the freezer and allow to partially thaw - about 5 minutes.
3 Blend in a food processor and serve immediately.

(Serves 4)

DRINKS AND SNACKS

The following drinks can be drunk without limit throughout
the day:
Water
Herb teas, such as Blackcurrant Bracer, Orange Dazzler and
          Apple Magic.
Coffee alternatives, such as Caro.

The following drinks are best limited to three glasses a day:
Aqua Libra
Fruit juices diluted 50 per cent with water

Limit alcohol to five units a week:
A glass of wine
A half pint of beer or lager
A measure of spirits

The only snacks allowed are two pieces of fruit each day choosing
from apples, bananas, oranges, pears, 6oz of grapes, or other more
exotic fruit of an equivalent size. Do not have more than one
banana per day as a snack. It is fine to have another banana in the
same day, if it is part of a recipe. It is best to have these snacks mid
morning and mid afternoon, away from your main meals.

SETTING YOUR TARGET & MONITORING YOUR PROGRESS

Most people start diets hoping to lose in a month what they gained in a year. They vow never to eat chocolate again and to exercise every day. This approach usually ends in failure.

Be Realistic

Our advice is to be realistic, and take it one step at a time. Set yourself targets for changing your diet and taking exercise that you know you will reach. The weight will look after itself. It is far better to take one step towards permanently changing your lifestyle, than to take four steps forward, and four steps back, on an over-ambitious regime.

After all, we often eat because we are under pressure or stressed. Boredom, frustration, anger, lack of direction all lead to feelings that can be temporarily suppressed with food. Even making small dietary changes is, to begin with, stressful. It takes time to adjust. So don't add to your stress by expecting too much from yourself and then failing to meet your targets.

Be Patient

You took years to get fat. Does it really matter if you take months, rather than weeks, to lose it? Our impatience drives us towards the countless 'get slim quick' diets that have been shown, time and time again, not to produce long-term results. It is very hard for the body to lose more than 1.5lbs in a week. 1.5lbs of body fat is about the same size as a brick. That's a lot of fat. More rapid weight loss is likely to be mainly the loss of short-term fluid. For example, when you eat too little carbohydrate for energy production, the body breaks down stores of glycogen. With every unit of glycogen nine units of water are lost. Instance weight loss. But once you increase your carbohydrate intake, the body will restore glycogen stores, plus the water.

A weight loss of 1lb a week, maintained over a year, equates to a loss of 3st 10lbs. This is easily achieved, without any suffering, on the Fatburner diet.

Don't forget that your body fat percentage is far more important than your weight. So don't rely on your scales as the only means for checking your progress. As you begin to make more lean muscle you won't lose so much weight, because lean muscle is heavier than the fat your burn off. But you will lose inches, since

Weight in pounds, wearing indoor clothing

Men of ages 25 and over		Women of ages 25 and over	
Height	Weight	Height	Weight
5' 1"	112-129	4' 8"	92-107
5' 2"	115-133	4' 9"	94-110
5' 3"	118-136	4' 10"	96-113
5' 4"	121-139	4' 11"	99-116
5' 5"	124-143	5' 0"	102-119
5' 6"	128-147	5' 1"	105-122
5' 7"	132-152	5' 2"	108-126
5' 8"	136-156	5' 3"	111-130
5' 9"	140-160	5' 4"	114-135
5' 10"	144-165	5' 5"	118-139
5' 11"	148-170	5' 6"	122-143
6' 0"	152-175	5' 7"	126-147
6' 1"	156-180	5' 8"	130-151
6' 2"	160-185	5' 9"	134-155
6' 3'	164-190	5' 10"	138-159

Figure 10 Your ideal weight

muscle is more compact than fat. Muscle cells are more metabolically active and therefore have the capacity to burn off fat, while fat cells don't. So, as you make more lean muscle, your ability to burn fat increases. Therefore, on the Fatburner approach, you'll be able to consistently lose weight and inches month after month.

Figure 10, on the previous page, shows your ideal weight range for your height. These figures are calculated from life insurance figures. If you're within your ideal range, we recommend that you don't aim to lose more than 4lbs a month, until you reach your target. If you are above the ideal range don't target to lose more than 6lbs a month.

Setting Your Target

When setting your target it is good to have long-term and short-term objectives. We call your long-term objective your goal. How you would, ideally, like to be. The following questions help to give you a realistic yardstick to go by. What do you weigh now? What is your ideal weight? When were you last that weight? What's the most you've ever lost on a diet?

Once you've set your long-term goal, which can be filled in on the Fatburner Progress Report on page 154, now work out your target, week by week. For example, if you want to lose 14lbs, your target after one week would be to weigh 2lbs less.

Monitoring Your Progress

Weigh and measure yourself at the beginning and end of every week. Always weigh yourself in the morning, before breakfast, without clothes. Keep monitoring your progress week after week. If you have a bad week notice what effect that has on your progress, and get back on course. If you reach a 'plateau' don't worry. This can happen. You can encourage weight loss to start again by following the Maximum Weight Loss tips on page 61 for two weeks. Soon, you'll find what you need to do to lose weight, and, once you've reached your ultimate goal, what you need to do to stay there.

Make some photocopies of the Fatburner Progress Report on page 154 (it's the one page we give you permission to copy) and fill it out for week one. You'll need an accurate pair of scales and a tape measure. Since scales do vary it's best to weigh yourself on the same scales each week. For the measurements always take the widest part of, for example, your thighs or your hips. For your thigh measurement take an average of your left and right thigh. (Either add the two measurements together and divide by two, or take the midway point, i.e. if the left thigh is 23 inches wide, and the right thigh is 21 inches wide, the average is 22 inches.) Your total inch loss is the sum of all the inches you have lost from measurements of your bust or chest, waist, hips and thighs. (If you've lost one inch from each your total inch loss is 4 inches.) Your target weight is your short term objective for this week. Your goal weight is your your long-term objective.

At the end of each week ask yourself, honestly, how well you've stuck to the diet and exercise programme. There's a space on the Progress Report to rate yourself out of 100%. This will help you to stay on course. If, at the end of the week you feel your targets are too hard or too easy you can adjust the rate of progress you're aiming for.

Get Fatburning now!

The FAT BURNER Progress Report

Full Name: _____ Membership No: _____

Tel No: _____ Best time to call: _____

Week No: [ ]   Starting date:__ /__ /__ Ending date: __ /__ /__

THIS WEEK

Initial Weight: _____ Bust: _____ Waist: _____ Hips: ____ Thighs: _____

Final Weight: _____ Bust: _____ Waist: _____ Hips: ____ Thighs: _____
(at end of week)

Target Weight: _____ Bust: _____ Waist: _____ Hips: ____ Thighs: _____

PROGRESS THIS WEEK

Weight Lost: _____ Total inch loss: _____

How many Air-obic Sessions?_____ How many Toning Sessions? _____

How well did you follow the diet? _____ %   the exercises? _____ %

PROGRESS TO DATE

Initial Weight: _____ Initial total inches: _____
(at start of diet)   (Bust + Waist + Hips + Thighs)

Weight Lost to date: _____ Inches lost to date: _____

© Patrick Holford 1992

USEFUL ADDRESSES

HEALTH+PLUS produce an extensive range of vitamin and mineral supplements available by mail order, including **The Metabolic Pack** and **Konjac Fibre**. Send for a free catalogue to: *Health+Plus, PO Box 86, Seaford, Sussex BN25 4ZW.*

THE INSTITUTE FOR OPTIMUM NUTRITION offers courses and personal consultations with qualified nutritionists, including Patrick Holford. On request ION will send you a free information pack. See page 159. *ION, 5 Jerdan Place, London SW6 1BE Tel: 071 385 7984; Fax: 071 385 3249.*

THE NUTRITION CONSULTANTS ASSOCIATION is an association of qualified nutrition consultants. They publish a directory of nutrition consultants throughout Great Britain which is available, either direct from them, or from ION for £1.50. *NCA c/o 5 Jerdan Place, London SW6 1BE.*

THE FATBURNER CLUB is a support club for fatburners. More details are given on page 158. For further details send an SAE to: *The Fatburner Club, PO Box 245, Weybridge, Surrey KT13 0YB.*

RECOMMENDED READING

Optimum Nutrition, *Patrick Holford* (ION Press) 1992, £4.95. The definitive guide to health and nutrition.

The Energy Equation, *Patrick Holford* (ION Press) 1988, £2.50. An in-depth look at energy and how to have more of it.

Supernutrition for a Healthy Heart, Patrick Holford (ION Press) 1989, £2.50. How heart disease develops, and what you can do combat it. Highly practical and informative.

How to Boost Your Immune System, *Jennifer Meek* (ION Press) 1988, £2.50. How the immune system works and how to boost it for relief from infections, allergies and immune diseases.

How to Improve Your Digestion and Absorption, *Christopher Scarfe* (available from ION Press) 1989, £2.50. A practical guide to improving the many problems of a poorly functioning digestive system.

How to Protect Yourself from Pollution, Patrick Holford & Dr. Philip Barlow (ION Press) 1990, £2.50. A crash course in the art of chemical self-defence.

Prices subject to alteration.
All these books are available, or can be ordered by your local health food shop.
They are also available, by mail order from ION.

INDEX

INDEX

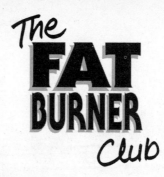

The FAT BURNER Club

Have you ever embarked on a diet and not stuck to it? Support is vital however determined you are to lose weight and get healthy. The Fatburner Club exists to give you that support every step of the way. Here's how:

As a member of the Fatburner Club you'll have:
- direct access to fatburning products, including vitamin supplements, Get Up & Go, the Fatburner exercise video, aerotubes, books, and any other vital supplies, at special prices.
- the opportunity to consult a qualified nutrition consultant in your area, trained in the Fatburner Diet approach, to give you personal advice (highly recommended for those who have difficulty losing weight).
- a telephone helpline giving you immediate support and a chance to have your fatburning questions answered.
- a week by week support system to keep you on target. information on 'fatburner approved' exercise classes in your area.
- regular updates on hot news such as new fatburning recipes, exercises, products, seminars, courses and ways of making weight control easier.
- a chance to participate in on-going fatburning research by the authors.

Membership is free. All you have to do is fill in the coupon below and send it to us, together with a large (A5 - 16x23cm) stamped and self addressed envelope.

— — — — — — — — — — — **A short cut to better health** — — — — — — — — — —

Mr, Ms _____ First Name _____ Surname _____

Address _____

County _____ Post Code _____

Your current weight: _____ Your ideal weight: _____

Phone Number: _____ Best time to call: _____

Now send this to: The FATBURNER Club, PO Box 245, Weybridge, Surrey KT13 0YB.

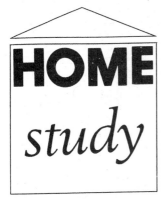

HOME *study*

Your car comes with a manual, but what about your body? Do you ever wonder what makes you tick? How you make energy from food? Why some people age faster than others? How to stay super healthy?

You'll find the answers in ION's Homestudy Course (that comes with 3 workbooks, 3 hours of video presentations, 12 taped lectures and step by step instructions to give you a solid grounding in optimum nutrition in 10 weeks.)

You'll learn more about nutrition than you thought possible - and have fun doing it, with practical homework, video presentations and taped lectures. The lecturers include many world authorities on nutrition. For example Professor Bryce-Smith will teach you how to protect yourself from pollution, Patrick Holford shows you how to promote vitality with vitamins and minerals, and Dr. Carl Pfeiffer teaches you how to prevent depression and improve memory.

Part 1 HOW YOUR BODY WORKS, teaches you how to improve digestion and absorption; balance nerves and hormones; and boost immune power. The second part, FOOD AND NUTRITION, looks at everything from the politics of food to wholefood cookery. You'll find out how to prevent heart disease and protect against cancer and arthritis, as well as learning how to detect your own allergies. In the final part, INDIVIDUAL NUTRITION, you'll learn how to work out individually tailored programmes. You'll find out all about nutrition for children and the elderly, as well as how to use nutrition for "first aid".

By the end of the course you'll know enough about nutrition to keep yourself and your family healthy. And you'll be able to help and advise your friends too.

When you enrol for the course you'll get all the course materials including the tapes, videos and workbooks which include written and practical homework for each section of the course.

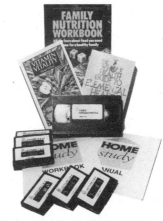

The course costs less than £10 a week, including all course material. Anyone can do it. All you need is a keen interest in nutrition.

A DETAILED PROSPECTUS IS AVAILABLE ON REQUEST

I. O. N.

The Institute for Optimum Nutrition is a non profit-making independent organisation that exists to help you promote your health through nutrition. ION was founded in 1984 and is based in London. ION offers educational courses starting with a one-day introductory course right up to a two year training to become a nutrition consultant; a clinic for one-to-one consultations; publications; and ION's magazine, Optimum Nutrition, which goes out free to members. If you'd like to receive more details please complete the details below.

Please send me your:

☐ FREE Information Pack
☐ Homestudy Course prospectus
☐ ION Clinic details
☐ Directory of Nutrition Consultants (enclose £1.50)

I'd like to order the following books: *(please list title, quantity & price)*

_____

_____

_____

_____

I enclose £ _____ payable to ION (Please add 10% for p&p)

First Name:_____ Surname: _____

Address:_____

_____

_____ Post Code: _____

Now send this to: ION, 5 Jerdan Place, London, SW6 1BE
(Tel:071 385 7984)